131
Ways
to live
131
Years

Dr. Valerie Walker

Brown Books Publishing Group
Dallas, Texas

131 Ways to live to 131 Years

Manufactured in the United States of America

Scriptures taken from the Holy Bible, New International Version®,
NIV®. Copyright © 1973, 1978, 1984 by Biblica, Inc.™
Used by permission of Zondervan. All rights reserved worldwide.
www.zondervan.com

For information please contact:
Brown Books Publishing Group
16200 North Dallas Parkway, Suite 170
Dallas, Texas 75248
www.brownbooks.com
(972) 381-0009

A New Era in Publishing™

ISBN-13: 978-1-934812-79-2
ISBN-10: 1-934812-79-X

LCCN: 2010934880
10 9 8 7 6 5 4 3 2 1

Author contact information:
www.DrValerieWalker.com

Dedicated to my father,
the Reverend Dr. James Albert Walker.

Contents

vii • Acknowledgments

ix • The Dirty Dozen

xi • The Body: An Overview

131 Ways

About the Author

Icon Key

Good Health

Nutrition

Physical Health

Mental Health

Acknowledgments

Special thanks to Chat Daniels—there are bankers, and then there's Chat Daniels! Thanks for believing in me and my dream.

To Carson D. Schneck, MD, PhD—probably the greatest anatomy professor of all time.

To Joseph Tollison, MD, and Joseph Hobbs, MD—both great physicians and great mentors from the Medical College of Georgia.

And also to the team at Brown Books Publishing Group. Thank you for all of your work.

The Dirty Dozen

The biggest offenders to one's healthy living:

1. Stress and anxiety

2. Saturated fats, trans fats, and high cholesterol

3. HPI (Habitual Physical Inactivity) and HMI (Habitual Mental Inactivity), which can lead to:
    - Obesity
    - Diabetes
    - Heart disease
    - High blood pressure
    - Alzheimer's disease

4. A potbelly with chicken legs (you junkaholic, you)

5. Smoking

6. Alcohol and illegal drugs

7. Paid character assassins

8. Social isolation and loneliness

9. Dehydration (most of you are dehydrated)

10. Sugar and other refined foods

11. The spirits: cheap, jealous, bitter, unforgiving

12. Pride . . . always comes before the fall

The Body: An Overview

I'm going to give you a quick overview of how the body works and how each bodily system functions.

Atoms, which provide the framework for all living activity, bond together to create molecules, which then form cells—the smallest functional unit on which all life is built. In order to perform the many diverse metabolic activities that occur within the body, each group of cells serves a specific function and communicates with one another to regulate growth and development. There are muscle cells, bone cells, and nerve cells, each of which is responsible for making up a different group of tissues in your body. Tissues are a group of similar cells performing a common function. For instance, your muscle tissue consists of *muscle* cells.

Tissues, then, form organs, which are made up of groups of different kinds of tissue working together to perform a specific activity. For example, your heart is an organ composed of muscle, connective, nerve, and epithelial tissues.

Next, we have organ systems, which are made up of two or more organs working together to accomplish a particular task. For instance, the digestive system involves the coordinated activities of many organs, including your mouth (you do have to chew your food, after all!), stomach, small and large intestine, liver, and pancreas.

Our bodies truly are amazing vessels for our spirits.

Now for a quick catalog of the bodily systems and their functions:

The circulatory system provides you with nutrients by bringing oxygen-rich blood to all areas of your body.

The digestive system actually starts with you seeing and salivating over that big, juicy hamburger. It then proceeds to the roots of your mouth and tongue and goes all the way down to the rectum, extracting nutrients from food and water and eliminating waste.

The endocrine system is responsible for hormone development, tissue function, puberty, and metabolism. This system includes your thyroid, pituitary, and adrenal glands, as well as the exocrine glands, which are responsible for the secretion of sweat, saliva, milk, and stomach acid.

The immune system is your own personal army. Just like those good-lookin' Navy SEALs can deliver a fatal blow with their bare hands, this system wards off any foreign invaders to the body including viruses, bacteria, parasites, and fungi.

The intergumentary system is probably the least talked-about system but is definitely just as important because it protects your body with gorgeous skin, which comes in a rainbow of beautiful colors. Skin also regulates temperature (that's why you sweat), vitamin D, and the excretion of salts and small amounts of water.

The muscular system involves all the muscles in your body, which work together with your bones and joints to help you stay mobile.

The nervous system is made up of all of your body's nerves including your brain and spinal cord. This system controls your thoughts, movement, temperature, sense, and ability to reason and think.

The reproductive system is where both pleasure and procreation take place. In the female, this system includes a pair of ovaries, the uterus, fallopian tubes, the cervix, and the vagina. In men, it includes the prostate gland, the penis, and a pair of testicles. Our reproductive system is capable of giving life and providing us with unbelievable pleasure at the same time—and that is nothing to be ashamed of!

The respiratory system brings oxygen to your body and removes carbon dioxide.

The sensory system includes your sense of sight, smell, taste, touch, and hearing. We're going to concentrate on how to maintain this system because it takes a lot of work!

The skeletal system is made up of all your bones, which allow you to stand tall and move around.

The urological system is made up of your kidneys, bladder, and urethra. Together these allow urine to pass from your body.

Together, these systems make up the incredible human body. Body systems are driven by numerous chemical reactions that occur in the body to keep you running like a well-oiled machine. Your body can be likened to a house because it, too, has electricity (literally), plumbing, gaseous exchange, walls, and a strong foundation that all work together to keep you alive.

Vitamins (necessary micronutrients), minerals, and trace elements all contribute to a healthy and long life, keeping the body under perfect control, or in "homeostasis." The human body has to be at peace with itself for optimal performance.

Now, let's begin our fabulous journey into living 131 years and beyond.

1

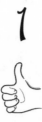

Know Your Family History

You can't run away from your DNA!

Grandma and Grandpa did the do and your mom and dad did, too—yuck! Whatever they've got, you might have, too. Diseases tend to run in families so you must stay informed and investigate your family history. You cannot afford to be a spectator when it comes to your health care. Come off the sidelines!

If things like heart disease, cancer, diabetes, depression, Alzheimer's, stroke, or any other disease run in your family, you've got to let your doctor know so he or she can start screening early and hopefully prevent some of these hereditary illnesses from affecting you.

Family history can help your doctor:
- Decide which medical tests to run
- Determine whether you would benefit from preventive measures to lower your risk of a specific disease
- Identify other members of your family who may be at risk of developing certain diseases
- Calculate your risk of passing certain conditions to your children
- Diagnose and calculate your risk for certain diseases

Even alcoholism can run in families. So help your doctor and be honest when he or she asks you how much you drink. Don't say you drink one beer every now and then when you know you're guzzling two six-packs every night. We see the bottles in the trash can—duh!

2

Drink Up

H₂0, that is . . .

H_2O, that is . . .

Divide your body weight in half and drink that amount of water in ounces each and every day. Don't want to drink that much? Then lose some weight, darling!

Did you know the human body is approximately 65 percent water? Next time you go out to eat and the server asks what you'd like to drink, avoid the sodas and cocktails and ask for water with lemon instead. You'll be doing something good for your body and your wallet. If you exercise daily like you're supposed to, always take a bottle of water with you. Sports drinks and energy drinks are full of carbohydrates, sugar, and calories (among other things), so they're not as good for you as plain old water. One of my elderly patients just told me the other day, "Sodas only make my mouth sweet and dry!"

Most people drink less than half the daily required amount of water for their body size. If you think I'm asking too much by telling you to drink water, you need to get over it because it doesn't get much easier than this. So get drinking—and I don't mean tequila! Water is beneficial in many ways. Obviously, it helps prevent dehydration. Dehydration often masquerades as hunger. It is very likely that the hunger pangs you're feeling are actually your body telling you it needs water. Proper hydration also helps your body:

- Prevent urinary tract infections
- Prevent kidney stones
- Prevent constipation
- Decrease fatigue
- Prevent some of those telltale signs of aging like crow's feet, wrinkles, and dry, sagging skin

Important:

If you have congestive heart failure, ESRD (end stage renal disease), or any disease where fluids are restricted, consult with your health-care professional about your water intake.

3

Eat Breakfast Every Day

Skipping breakfast isn't going to help you lose weight.
So go ahead and enjoy the breakfast of champions.

A lot of people skip breakfast in the morning for a variety of reasons. Some say they are trying to lose weight, others say they aren't hungry first thing in the morning, and some say they simply don't have enough time to eat before work. This is just like running your car on empty. You aren't going to get very far with an empty gas tank, and your body is no different. Remember how your grandmother always used to tell you breakfast is the most important meal of the day? Well, guess what—Grandma was right! I can't stress to you how important it is that you get up fifteen minutes early each day so you can sit down and eat a nutritious breakfast. That's right—I said nutritious. Skip the doughnuts and sugary cereals and try oatmeal with whole-grain toast instead.

People who think they aren't affected by not eating breakfast are sadly mistaken. Going without nourishment until lunchtime causes your blood sugar to drop drastically, which will leave you with a headache and a sluggish, hostile, fatigued feeling. Maybe that's why you're screaming at all your coworkers. Girl, you're hungry! Have fun explaining to your boss why you didn't meet your deadline! To make matters worse, you'll be so hungry at lunchtime you will most likely eat more food, and it's more likely to be the wrong food, laden with fat. This will lead to weight gain—just the opposite of what you were going for.

One of the first steps to living 131 years is to start each morning with a well-balanced meal that will nourish your body, give you energy, and help you stay focused all day long. Regardless of when your day starts (even if you're a shift worker), make sure you eat your breakfast. My favorite breakfast is sautéed mushrooms, spinach, and some low-fat cheese scrambled with egg whites. Delicious—try some!

Brush Your Teeth and Tongue

Good morning, Sunshine! Don't even think about leaving your house in the morning without brushing your teeth and that nasty tongue! Bad breath is not appealing.

Do you know someone who has no sense of personal space and always has to be right up in your face when they're talking to you? I find it funny that these always seem to be the same people who have the worst breath on Earth. Seriously, I've smelled some breath that could be classified as a weapon of mass destruction. Call Homeland Security!

Did you know mushroom-shaped stalks called papillae cover the surface of your tongue? Well, they do, and a lot of odor-producing, decaying food particles and bacteria can hide here. Brushing alone does not always remove these particles—you've got to scrape them off. The best tool for that is a tongue scraper, which can be purchased at your local pharmacy for around five dollars and is very simple to use. The goal is to clean that crap off your tongue and keep your breath fresh and oral hygiene on point.

Do your mouth (and the population at large) a favor and brush your teeth and tongue at least twice each day. If you want to go the extra mile and brush between meals, floss, and gargle with mouthwash, then I applaud your dedication to fresh breath and oral hygiene! Remember: when it comes to mouthwash, once in the morning does it! You should brush for at least two minutes and replace your toothbrush every two to three months and after recovering from an illness. Don't let the toothbrush patrol catch you with that raggedy toothbrush!

It's not just your pearly whites that make your smile so fabulous. It's also knowing you're not swallowing all that bacteria in your mouth that some research suggests can cause numerous medical diseases. For instance, did you know that dental cavities and poor oral hygiene have been linked to heart disease and cancer?

5

Get Plenty of Quality Sleep

Stay out of bed unless you're sleeping, sick, or having sex.

The average adult needs approximately eight hours of sleep each night, and young people need even more. Your bedroom should be a haven for a good night's sleep—make it a tropical oasis! The ideal sleep environment is a dark, cool, quiet room. Try earplugs to drown out environmental noise or play white noise if you need help unwinding. Have you ever wondered why hotel rooms are so relaxing? It's because there are no distractions and no clutter! Your bedroom should be the same way. By the way, a big part of this is cleaning up your bedroom. Why do you have that big pile of dirty, smelly clothes in the corner of your bedroom? And then you call me at 3 a.m. saying you can't sleep. That makes two of us. Goodnight, sleep tight! Your body has routine repairs to make!

You also shouldn't be hanging out in your bedroom playing on your laptop, reading a book, or staring at bills you know you can't pay. Your bed is for sleeping in, not hanging out, talking on the phone, or watching television. Avoid doing the three T's (talking, texting, and television) in your bedroom. Stay out of there unless you're doing one of the three S's (sleeping, being sick, or having sex).

If you want to get a good night's sleep, heavy meals before bedtime are not a good idea. Have a glass of warm milk or a piece of fruit instead. You should also try going to bed at the same time every night and getting up at the same time each morning. Yes, even on the weekend! Eventually your body will adapt to this pattern and you will find yourself going to bed and waking up at about the same time every day without even trying. This is called the circadian rhythm—your body's internal alarm clock. Soon you'll find yourself in a better mood, feeling more rested, and accomplishing more throughout the day. My patients always tell me they like to sleep in or catch up on sleep on the weekend. I don't think so. It doesn't work that way! So, if you have extra time on Saturday morning, hallelujah! You can get up and exercise. And if you have time on Sunday morning, go to church! The best sleeping pill is peace of mind.

6

Exercise Regularly

Get off the couch, step away from the computer, and put on your tennis shoes.

Having a regular exercise routine that you stick to is imperative to good health. Did you know the best exercise is consistency? Pick something you like and stick with it. Personally, I've always been a walker. My morning walks are how I clear my head, plan out my day, and have some quiet time to myself before work. Even in the middle of winter, I bundle up and go out for my morning walk. Unless the ground is covered in ice, my morning routine is pretty much the same year-round. God gave you feet and legs for a reason, so get off the couch! Remember, Jesus walked almost everywhere for the brief thirty-three years he was here. Regardless of how old you are, walking is great exercise. Even old folks can get up, walk four feet forward, turn around, and go back with assistance—so no excuses! In addition to walking, I also exercise with Charley Johnson at Charley's Body Shop here in St. Louis. Always keep in mind that variety is the spice of life.

Before you start exercising, invest in a good pair of walking shoes that bend at the toe. Don't buy shoes thinking you're going to break them in! Ill-fitting shoes are thought to be the cause of 80 percent of all foot-related problems. And don't forget to stretch before and after your walk. Girl, don't tell me the last time you stretched was when you gave birth. Don't be an exercise weekend warrior—you will go down in battle!

Exercise has so many benefits. It improves your cardiovascular health, increases endorphins (those feel-good chemicals your body produces), and helps you maintain a healthy weight. There are many ways to get your blood pumping including team sports, swimming, water aerobics, Jazzercise, stepaerobics, and weight training—just to name a few. If all else fails, go dancing!

Exercise also helps relieve anxiety and depression symptoms, and it can even help you sleep better at night. I encourage you to jump on the fitness bandwagon because this is one trend I can't imagine ever going out of style.

7

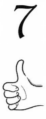

Stop Smoking

And tell your smoking spouse to keep their butt outside!

Smoking is terrible for your health, so it's no wonder that it's the number one preventable cause of death. Did you know cigarette smoke contains over four thousand chemicals including tar, nicotine, arsenic, and carbon monoxide? The hazardous health effects of exposure to tobacco products (including cigars, snuff of all flavors, and chewing tobacco) are now well documented. There is no doubt within the international scientific community that smoking is linked to heart disease, lung cancer, nasal sinus cancer, sudden infant death syndrome, asthma, and ear infections in children.

Secondhand smoke (also known as passive smoke or enviro-nmental tobacco smoke) is just as bad for you, and the people around you, as smoking a cigarette firsthand. Secondhand smoke exposure is associated with strokes, low birth weight, miscarriages, negative effects on the development of cognitive behavior, exacerbation of cystic fibrosis, and cervical cancer.

Remember the Marlboro Man? He died of cancer!

Prevent exposure:
- Don't allow others to smoke in your home or car. Remove ashtrays from both.

- Sit in the nonsmoking section in restaurants.
- When people ask me, "Do you mind if I smoke?" I reply with, "Do you mind if I die?"
- If you smoke, set a date to quit and ask your health-care provider for help.

Fact:

The Family Smoking Prevention and Tobacco Control Act, which was signed by President Barack Obama, granted the FDA the authority to oversee tobacco products. Under the new law, the agency will establish standards for tobacco products and establish and enforce marketing restrictions.

8

Don't Be an Unforgiving Spirit

When someone does you wrong, that's not between you and them, it's between them and God. Let Him deal with them while you take the high road!

Has anyone ever done something to you that you can't seem to let go? I know I've experienced this in my own life. Everyone has probably yelled the famous words "I'll never forgive you!" at some point in their lives. I think the main reason we do this is because we don't really understand what it means to forgive. Forgiving someone is 100 percent about you and allowing yourself to move on. Forgiveness has nothing to do with excusing someone's hateful words or actions—absolutely nothing.

When you hold on to something, you let it get the best of you. So don't let the past take all of your valuable time and energy. Look forward and concentrate on the people and things that deserve your attention. Let God deal with those who have hurt you; they can answer to Him at the end of the day.

The best way to move on is to stop talking about it and thinking about it. Holding a grudge is like ripping the scab off a sore that's trying to heal. Every time you bring up those bad memories, the healing process has to start over again. We must forgive because God has a forgiving spirit, and who knows better than He? Our Lord forgives all of the transgressions that we commit against Him daily.

Just like Grandma used to say, "Let sleeping dogs lie!"

9

Stay Positive

Instead of wallowing in negativity and despair, take action to make your life lighter and brighter.

We've all had our bad days in this life. Shoot, some of us have had bad weeks, months, or even years! We all deal with this differently. Not everyone has the resilience to bounce back from a crisis after a short period of time. Some people crumble under pressure and some people prevail. That's OK. What you don't want to do is let the dark periods in your life leave you pessimistic and jaded. Instead, stay positive by counting three things every day that you're grateful for.

Have you ever noticed it's much easier to be negative than to look on the bright side of things? Smiling on a rainy day takes effort, but remember that flowers bloom after the rain. Smiling and thinking positive thoughts can have a profound effect on your life. Try being an optimist for a week and see how everything starts to fall into place for you.

Some people go through life being a victim. I call this the poor me syndrome. "I don't have a man, a house, a car, or money!" Well, guess what, if you're reading this book, you at least have your sight. That's something! Quit being a victim and embrace the day. Studies suggest that people who stay positive and see the glass half full instead of half empty live longer, more fulfilling lives. And don't invite me to your pity party . . . because I'm not coming. We all love to say "Life ain't fair." Correct. Life ain't fair! It hasn't been fair since Adam and Eve, so stop complaining.

- "I don't have the investment skills of Warren Buffet!"—Get over it!
- "I can't interview like Oprah!"—Few can!
- "I don't have a technological mind like Bill Gates!"—I don't either!

Enjoy your life wherever you are right now—it's where you're supposed to be.

10

Have a Plan

*It's up to you to have the guts and determination
to make your life exciting.*

Obviously you can't plan out every detail in life; there are far
too many variables to consider. There's something to be said for
spontaneity, too. What fun would life be if you had every moment
planned out and calculated? Not much, probably. But I do think it's
wise to have some sort of basic idea as to where you're headed and
how you're going to get there. It's important to stretch yourself in
order to change and become a better person. Everyone needs to set
goals for themselves to encourage personal growth. What's going on
tomorrow? What about a year from now? Where do you want to be
in five years? You do not want to die with your dreams left inside
you, so stop procrastinating! Just remember: unless you're the lead
sled dog, the view never changes.

A great tool that I encourage my patients to use is a dream
board. Basically, you take a big poster board and paste a picture of
yourself in the middle. Around your picture, paste photos of things
that represent what you want for yourself in the near future. Need
a new car? Find a picture of the exact car you want and paste it on
your board. This visual tool can work wonders.

Tips for goal-setting:

- Make a dream board.
- Write out your daily goals each morning, plan how you're going to get them done, and move toward them!
- Write out your goals for next year or five years from now. Make a plan of action and get started!

Never put off 'til tomorrow what you can do today. Don't keep telling me you're going to lose one hundred pounds next year. Start now! I cannot stress to you enough the urgency of now.

11

Prevent Heart Disease

Keep your heart happy and healthy!

Coronary heart disease (also called CHD) refers to the narrowing of the small blood vessels that supply blood and oxygen to your heart. Symptoms of CHD include chest pain or pressure (angina) or pain in the sternum, neck, arms, back, or even the jaw (this can feel like a toothache). You may also experience a feeling like someone is squeezing your heart, shortness of breath, and/or fatigue. Some people just report feeling an impending sense of doom.

Heart disease can be caused by many things, including plaque buildup in your arteries (usually from eating too many fatty foods), diabetes, high blood pressure, smoking, lack of exercise, alcohol abuse, kidney disease, and, of course, genetics.

Here are some steps you can take to help prevent heart disease:
- Don't smoke!
- Eat well-balanced meals.
- Exercise regularly, at least thirty minutes per day.
- Keep your cholesterol and blood sugar under control.
- Limit your saturated fat intake.
- Reduce stress in your life.
- Laugh a lot. Even God had a sense of humor—He made us!
- Maintain your ideal body weight.

- Keep your blood pressure at a healthy level, ideally at around 120/80.
- Stay away from drugs and limit alcohol intake.

Fact:

Heart disease is the leading cause of death for both men and women in the United States.

12

Guard against Diabetes

How sweet it isn't.

Diabetes is a serious disease that can be hereditary. It develops when your body doesn't produce enough insulin or respond to insulin in a normal way. Insulin is a hormone produced by your pancreas that controls the body's glucose levels by helping your body's cells use it for nourishment and energy. Glucose is a sugar that is converted in the body from the food you eat. Diabetes is diagnosed when your doctor sees that your body's blood glucose levels are too high.

Risk factors for developing diabetes include: family history, not getting enough exercise, being overweight, and even being of a specific ethnicity. Symptoms include lack of energy, frequent urination, vision problems, weight loss, and/or excessive thirst or hunger. With diabetes you may be eating and drinking constantly and still losing weight. You can help prevent diabetes by exercising daily, staying at your ideal body weight, eating healthy food, and controlling your blood pressure.

You should also know the diabetes ABCs:
- HBAIc: This test determines how high your blood glucose level is. It should be less than 7, but I like more stringent control with my patients and try to keep them at 6.5 or less.

- Blood pressure: Ideally 120/80 or lower.
- Cholesterol: Keep your HDL high and LDL low.
- Diet: watch what you eat!
- Exercise.

As part of your closely monitored diet, limit your alcohol intake. Watch your carbohydrates; older patients tend to tell me that they don't know why their sugar is high because they don't eat pie or cake. But did you know that carbohydrates can send your sugar levels soaring? And heaven forbid you eat that half of a watermelon; you'll surely enjoy it, but it can send your sugar through the roof. Stick with the plan! Monitor your carbohydrate intake.

Fact:

Diabetics who smoke are three times more likely to die of heart disease than those who do not.

13

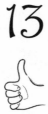

Know the Seven Warning Signs of Cancer

Pay attention to your body when your body is talking to you.

Cancer is the uncontrolled growth of abnormal cells in the body. Cancerous cells are also called malignant cells.

Your body should run like a well-oiled machine. When it's not, it can sometimes warn you that things are going awry, and it is not at peace with itself. When that happens, it's time to find out why.

The seven warning signs of cancer:
- Sores that do not heal.
- Bleeding from the rectum.
- Moles that change in asymmetry, border, color, and/or diameter.
- A persistent cough, especially if you are a smoker.
- Unusual vaginal bleeding and/or discharge. Ladies, if your doctor has diagnosed you as menopausal and you start to have vaginal bleeding again, this is not the rebirth of your childbearing years. Call your doctor!
- Discharge from the nipple/breast or a lump in the breast.
- A sore throat that will not heal or trouble swallowing.

If you develop *any* of these symptoms, you must notify your doctor immediately. When making an appointment, be sure to let the secretary know your symptoms and concerns. Don't delay; these symptoms may not go away. I can't stress this enough: Early detection! Early detection! Early detection! Remember, an ounce of prevention is worth a pound of cure.

14

Always Buckle Up Kids (and Yourself) for Safety

I don't care if you don't like seatbelts—
they can save your life!

Many deaths involving children in automobile accidents could have been prevented by properly securing children with seatbelts and car seats.

One of the easiest ways to prevent injury in a motor vehicle is to wear your seatbelt and ensure that all children are properly secured. You should also know whether your child needs a car seat and ensure they have the proper one. Here are some general guidelines to follow:

- Rear-facing seats: Use these in the backseat from newborn to at least one year old, or twenty pounds. It is safest to keep your baby rear-facing as long as possible, up to the weight limit of your rear-facing convertible seat. This should be around thirty or thirty-five pounds.
- Forward-facing toddler seats: Use these in the backseat from age one and twenty pounds to about age four and forty pounds. It is safest to keep your child in a five-point harness as long as possible, taking into account the upper weight limit of the seat.
- Booster seats: Use these in the backseat from about age four and forty pounds to at least eight years old, or until your child is 4'9".

- Safety belts: Transition to using only a safety belt at eight years old, or when your child is taller than 4'9".

Make sure you read all directions and safety warnings from the manufacturer of your car seat.

I see a lot of children pleading with their parents to sit in the front seat. Children are naturally curious, and they want to be grown up and have a better view like Mom and Dad. Remember, the backseat is the safest place for all kids under eight years old. And adults, it goes without saying, but wear your seatbelts as well—even if you're only going a short distance. Most accidents happen close to home.

15

Get Your Moles Checked

Keep an eye out for changes in symmetry, border, color, and diameter.

I can't stress this enough: If you have moles that are changing in shape, color, or size, get them checked immediately by your health-care provider. Changes in moles can be a sign of malignant melanoma, which often occurs near an existing mole and is one of the deadliest forms of skin cancer. Skin cancer is fatal and can spread rapidly to other organs.

Even if you notice changes, never try removing a mole yourself. Put that string down—I see you! Go see your doctor.

Have a full-body mole check by your health-care provider once a year, and check your own moles regularly for changes with the mole ABCs.

- Asymmetry: A mole should be a mirror image of itself. Is one half unlike the other? Imagine a line going down the center of a new pencil eraser. Like your moles, it should look the same on both sides.
- Border: Is the border poorly defined?
- Color: Is the color uneven or changing?
- Diameter: Is the mole bigger than the head of a pencil eraser or growing?

Early in my career, my first patient with malignant mela-noma was a twenty-eight-year-old sailor from California who enjoyed being in the sun without using sunscreen. Damage from the sun accumulated over time and unfortunately, at the time of diagnosis, his cancer had already begun to spread.

16

Always Wear Sunscreen

*Wear a sunscreen of SPF 15 or more every day,
even if you're African-American.*

There are two types of ultraviolet (UV) radiation—UVA and UVB. They both damage the skin and increase your risk for developing skin cancer. UVB rays cause sunburn. UVA rays penetrate your skin more deeply and cause skin to look wrinkled, saggy, and leathery. Sexy, huh? This is also referred to as photo-aging. UVA rays also assist UVB rays in damaging your skin and causing skin cancer—a double whammy! Sunscreen is a chemical agent that helps prevent the sun's UV radiation from getting to your skin and damaging it.

Also, keep in mind that although some sunshine is healthy and necessary to boost vitamin D levels, you should avoid direct sun between 11 a.m. and 3 p.m. Using sunscreen and limiting exposure are the best ways to prevent both damage to your skin and skin cancer itself. SPF (sun protection factor) is a measure of a sunscreen's ability to prevent UVB rays from damaging your skin. Sunscreen with an SPF of 15 or higher does a great job of protecting against UVB rays.

To make sure you get the full benefits of sunscreen, you need to apply at least one ounce to all sun-exposed areas. To be most effective, sunscreen must be applied thirty minutes prior to sun exposure to give it time to fully bind to the skin. Reapply the same amount every two hours and immediately after swimming, toweling off, or sweating during exercise.

I remember my grandma picking flowers with her apron, long-sleeved shirt, and wide-brimmed hat on. She knew what she was doing! On a personal note, when I go to the beach clad in my skimpy bikini (just kidding . . . actually, no, I wasn't), I always slather on my sunscreen—much to the delight of fellow beachgoers!

17

Try Yoga

Yoga isn't just for New Age junkies anymore.
This ancient practice benefits the body, mind, and spirit.

Looking for a great way to exercise that can calm the mind, relax the body, and help increase flexibility and muscle growth? Yoga involves a collection of techniques where you hold your body in a series of positions for set amounts of time to increase flexibility and physical strength. These techniques and practices aim at integrating mind, body, and spirit to achieve a state of enlightenment and unity with the universe. They can also help you overcome obstacles in your health.

There are several different styles of yoga that emphasize different approaches and techniques, but they ultimately have the same goal of unifying the mind, body, and spirit. Hatha is the style most practiced in the United States. The only supplies you need to start practicing yoga are some form-fitting clothes, a yoga mat, and plenty of water to stay hydrated during your workout.

Yoga therapists might suggest physical postures to develop balanced strength, flexibility (pranayama) to optimize your flow of breath, and meditation or reflection to help focus your understanding of the source of tensions that contribute to your symptoms.

I remember my first yoga class. I exercised so vigorously at Charley's Body Shop doing aerobics and stepaerobics that I thought yoga would be a breeze! Holding and maintaining a pose on a mat? OK! But the instructor nearly killed me, and I definitely worked up a sweat! I've been in love with yoga ever since.

To find a yoga therapist, you can contact the International Association of Yoga Therapists by visiting their website at www. IAYT.org. Take a friend and try something new!

18

Find Inner Happiness

Don't look to people, places, or things (the nouns!)
to make you happy. Happiness is an inside job.

O ur happiness always seems to be predicated on something outside of ourselves. So often I hear people say, "I'd be happy if I had a better job," or "I'd be happy if I had a good man." My personal favorite is, "I'd be happy if I had more money." Well, I hate to burst your bubble, but like I always say, "Money only affords you a new brand of misery."

You have all the tools you need to be happy in this world. Stop playing the blame game. If you want to know what's wrong with your life, go look in the mirror! Quit looking outside yourself for happiness and, instead, find peace within. Medication isn't always the answer, and you owe it to yourself to work on yourself before trying a pill. So whistle while you work!

Volunteer, feed the hungry, spend time with an elderly person, and practice random acts of kindness. If the carts at your supermarket require a twenty-five cent deposit, give your cart to the next shopper and make someone's day. You can derive much happiness from doing for others. Take a homebound senior to the park and feed the ducks. Happy people are fun to be around—like myself! They have all this positive energy flowing around them that would rub off on you if you'd stop being such a sourpuss! So go ahead and smile, you're on the world's candid camera.

19

Remember: Pride Comes Before the Fall

Newsflash: You are not the center of the universe!

Are you a proud, boisterous person basking in your own vanity, thinking the only reason the sun shines is because of you? Think about it—have you noticed that the bigger people get in their own minds and in the eyes of the world, the more problems they seem to have? There should always be little "i" and big "U."

> *"Pride goes before destruction, a haughty spirit before a fall."*
> *—Proverbs 16:18*

Take a step back and realize that you are not the center of the universe. Selfishness and vanity will only lead to self-destruction and misery in the long run. Don't let this happen to you! Be all you can be in this life, but stay humble and sincere. You never have to try putting someone else's candle out to make your light shine brighter. God wants you to use your vast potential, so go ahead—aspire to greatness, but never forget who the real boss is! Avoid bragging about yourself and looking down on others who are not as fortunate as you. I know people who will not attend an event unless they are given front row seats in the center. Quit whining, and be grateful for what you have. Remember, it could all be taken away in an instant.

Stay humble. Stay sincere.

"Woe to those who are wise in their own eyes
and clever in their own sight."
—Isaiah 5:21

20

Get Your Eyes Checked Regularly

I see you, but can you see me?

Many people feel that since they don't have any obvious problems with their vision, they don't need to go to the eye doctor. Wrong! You might have something wrong with your eyes and not even know it until it's too late. Regardless of your age, it's entirely possible that you could wake up one morning and not even be able to see your glasses peeping right back at you on the nightstand! Cataracts could be forming on your eyes right now, and you don't even know it. Everyone needs an eye exam—even young people. And if you're moving your paper back and forth to see better, it may be time to get your eyes checked!

You should be seeing an optometrist at least once a year to have your vision and pressures checked. If you have a family history of glaucoma, it is important that you let your doctor know so he or she can check regularly for elevated pressure in your eyes. If you don't have an eye doctor, ask your health-care provider for a referral.

You should always select an eye-care specialist with the correct training to meet your individual needs. If you have serious vision problems, you should see an ophthalmologist. For more common vision problems, or if you just need a prescription for corrective lenses or contacts, you should see a doctor of optometry.

When my patients don't remember how important their vision is, I tell them to close their eyes, look around the room, and tell me what they see. Everyone needs their eyesight, even young people. I remember getting my first pair of glasses when I was six years old. The teacher sat me in the back of the classroom because I was so tall and told my mother she noticed me squinting trying to see the board.

You need your peepers! In addition to seeing an eye doctor, eat food with vitamin A—it's great for your eyes. It can be found in carrots, milk, liver (I'll let you have that one), eggs, and cheese.

21

Read!

You couldn't wait to learn to read when you were a child and now you can't be bothered. What happened?

I am a firm believer in exercising the brain, especially because it may help ward off certain forms of dementia such as Alzheimer's. You know what they say—use it or lose it! Reading is an excellent way to keep your mind sharp, stay informed, and stay out of trouble. When was the last time you read a book just for fun? I'm not talking about something for work or school; I mean something that was actually enjoyable to read. Like this book, for example!

There are so many wonderful books, magazines, and newspapers available to us. Instead of flipping on the television or getting on the Internet when you get home from work or school, try sitting down in your favorite chair with a good book and reading for an hour or so. You'll be amazed at how fun reading can be. Just don't fall asleep!

If you have children, read to them at least twenty minutes every day. Some of my favorite memories from my childhood are of my mother or father reading to me as I drifted off to sleep. I felt so special. Don't let your child's education come exclusively from television—read, read, read!

If you're feeling charitable, read to someone who can't read for themselves. Volunteer at a nursing home or hospital, read for children, or even read to your own grandparents. Sometimes it's easy to forget how lucky we are to live in the United States where we are able to go to school and learn to read. Let's not take this luxury for granted.

For more information, visit www.reading.org.

22

Stop Lying

The truth will haunt you.

Like Judge Judy says, "You've got to have a good memory to be a liar." Every time you lie, the story changes a little bit. But the truth remains the same. Satan is the father of all lies—that's why he was relegated to a pit! Pits are where snakes and spiders reside. Does that sound like somewhere you want to be hanging out?

When people get in trouble for lying, they seem to always say, "I just told a little white lie!" There is no such thing as a little white lie! When did it become little? And by all means, explain to me how it became white. Inquiring minds want to know! I've met some pretty smooth talkers in my lifetime, but few have been able to pull the wool over these eyes. As the Bible says, "The truth shall set you free." We should all aspire to an honest lifestyle, free of deception and lies. You see, there is no right way to do a wrong thing. Enough said.

Consequences of lying:
- Lying can ruin your relationships.
- It will make you nervous and afraid because you don't know when the truth is going to come out—and it will come out! What's done in the night will always come to light.

- It will give you restless and sleepless nights.

"Let their lying lips be silenced."
—Psalms 31:18

23

Install and Maintain
Smoke Detectors

Don't let your safety go up in smoke!

Did you know that most fire victims die from the inhalation of smoke and toxic gases, not from burns? The majority of these deaths occur at night when victims are asleep and don't notice the fire. Having smoke detectors properly installed and maintained in your home is one of the best and least expensive ways to prevent these kinds of deaths. Smoke detectors save lives, prevent injuries, and minimize damage to homes by alerting residents to fires early in their development.

Fire safety is an easy way to save lives. Simply install, test, and maintain smoke detectors in your home, and practice a fire escape plan. All smoke detectors in your house should be tested monthly, and batteries should be replaced annually. Your family should also develop a fire escape plan and practice it at least twice a year.

A few years ago, one of my friends had the man she was seeing over for a home-cooked dinner. Well, she shouldn't have lied and said she knew how to cook because she forgot about the roast in the oven. When her date finally arrived, she was trying to get all of the smoke out of the house. I don't think she saw much of him after that night, but at least the smoke detectors kept her safe.

Facts:

- You are twice as likely to die in a fire in a home without smoke detectors.
- Deaths from fires and burns are the fifth most common cause of unintentional injury death in the United States.
- Four out of five fire deaths in the United States occur in private homes.
- Every year in the United States, approximately three thousand people lose their lives in residential fires.

24

Get a Second Opinion

You can never be too careful with your health.

Medicine is an art. Even though doctors receive similar medical training, each will have his or her own unique style and flair that they bring to their practice. Different doctors have different ideas about how to best diagnose, approach, and treat diseases and medical conditions while still maintaining high standards of quality care. Some of the old doctors out in the country, which is where I grew up, would make a strange concoction right there in the office and tell you to drink it—and you actually felt better! Then you have doctors like me, who practice spiritual, holistic, and traditional medicine all in one visit.

Getting a second opinion about a grave diagnosis from a different doctor might give you a new perspective and different information. This can help you decide what path to take regarding treatment, especially if you still have doubts and/or concerns. More knowledge allows you to make more informed choices. If you have a major decision to make about your body and your health, don't have shame in your game!

Here are some tips for getting a second opinion if you are uncomfortable with the diagnosis and/or treatment that you are receiving, or if you just want to know more:

- Check with your health insurance provider to make sure a second opinion will be covered by your insurance. They can also provide a referral.
- Ask your doctor for a recommendation. We're tough, we can handle it! Don't worry about hurting your doctor's feelings. Getting a second opinion is not uncommon in the medical field.
- Ask someone you trust, like a friend or a family member, for a recommendation.
- Ask to have all medical records sent to the second doctor.
- Learn as much as you can about your condition. Do your own research so you know what questions to ask.

25

Be Aware of Suicide Warning Signs

Don't be afraid to ask for help.

In 2006, suicide was the eleventh leading cause of death in the United States, accounting for 33,300 deaths. Know the warning signs and, if you recognize them in yourself or others, seek help immediately.

What to look for:
- Suicidal ideation: thinking about, talking about, or wishing for death/suicide
- Substance use or abuse, especially increased use of, or change in, substances
- Purposelessness: feeling no real sense of purpose or belonging
- Frequent mood changes and anger
- Feeling trapped, like there's no way out
- Hopelessness: feeling like there is nothing to live for, no hope, and no cause for optimism
- Withdrawal from family, friends, work, school, activities and/or hobbies
- Recklessness: high risk-taking behavior

There is always hope, regardless of what you're going through. Remember, God has a plan for your life.

To contact a crisis center call the National Suicide Prevention Lifeline at 1-800-273-TALK

Facts:

Women are more likely to attempt suicide and survive. Men are less likely to attempt suicide but more likely to succeed when they do.

26

Get a Massage

Get one—it's not kinky anymore!

Do you want to feel invigorated, emancipated, and rejuven-ated? Look no further than a relaxing massage. Find yourself a licensed massage therapist, one who graduated from an accredited school of massage therapy, and indulge yourself!

Benefits of massage:
- Deep tissue release
- Improved circulation
- Relief from joint stiffness
- Reduction in blood pressure
- Alleviated stress
- Improved lymphatic flow

You should incorporate massage into your wellness package as much as your budget will allow. All massage techniques are not created equally. There are Swedish massages, shiatsu, sports, and many more. Try them all until you find the one that's right for you! Deep tissue is my personal favorite, but this can be pretty intense and involve a lot of pressure, so check with your health-care provider before making an appointment.

Be sure to drink plenty of water after a massage to wash away toxins that have built up and get released during and after your session. Relax and get a massage—you deserve it!

For more information or to find a massage therapist in your area, visit www.amtamassage.org.

27

Trigger Your Endorphins

It's a natural high!

Ever wonder what makes you feel happy? Why is it that you feel so much better after a long run, making love to your spouse, or having a good laugh with your girlfriends? That high feeling, which can last up to twelve hours (or even more for some people), has a scientific explanation: It comes from the release of endorphins in your body.

Endorphins are morphine derivatives and neurotransmitters (chemicals that relay signals between cells) that block the reuptake of the serotonin produced in your brain. They reduce pain, elevate your mood, and make you feel fabulous all over. When you exercise or exert energy in some way, these endorphins are released into your system. Some studies show that positive thinking alone is enough to trigger the release of endorphins. How powerful is that?

Ways to trigger endorphins:
- Exercise
- Have sex (with your spouse, of course!)
- Think positive thoughts
- Laugh
- Eat foods like dark chocolate (yum!) and chili peppers

So how many endorphins can you stand to release? Go find out! But don't go telling everyone I told you to sit in the middle of your bed eating dark chocolate, thinking positive thoughts, and waiting for some endorphins to be released! Remember that the bedroom is your oasis for sleep!

28

Recognize that We Are Living in Perilous Times

Talk to God—crying to each other does no good.

"This know also, that in the last days perilous times shall come."

Read 2 Timothy 3:1–17. This is where the apostle Paul is speaking to his young preacher, Timothy. These are perilous times. Domestic violence, gang wars, assaults, incest, child molestation, burglaries, storms, hurricanes, murders, terrorist attacks, suicides, genocides, homicides, wars, and rumors of war. These things happen around us all day, every day.

So, I know you're asking now, "What should we be doing?" Go to I Kings 2:1–3 in the Old Testament where King David, the second king of Israel, is speaking to his son Solomon and giving him the instruction to "Keep God's commandments as it is written in the law of Moses, that thou mayest prosper in all that thou doest, and withersoever thou turnest thyself."

The Ten Commandments (Exodus 20:1–17):
- Thou shalt have no other gods before me.
- Thou shalt not make unto thee any graven image.
- Thou shalt not take the name of the Lord thy God in vain.

- Remember the Sabbath day to keep it holy.
- Honor thy father and thy mother.
- Thou shalt not kill.
- Thou shalt not commit adultery.
- Thou shalt not steal.
- Thou shalt not bear false witness against thy neighbor.
- Thou shalt not covet thy neighbor's house.

What part of "thou shalt not" do you not understand?

The power of prayer can't be explained by science, but it definitely works. I promise. Pray without ceasing. And remember, don't look around—look up.

29

Prevent Work-Related Injuries and Deaths

Slow down, fool! Take care while doing dangerous work.

In 2007, 5,657 work-related fatalities were reported in the United States. You don't want to become a statistic—be aware of any dangerous tasks that are part of your job, and be careful when undertaking them.

Tips for preventing injury and death on the job:
- Educate yourself. Take the time to learn all important safety information for the job you do. If you work with dangerous chemicals or machines, you should know what to do if something is spilled or is not operating correctly. If you have questions, ask a supervisor.
- Use proper safety equipment, including protective head gear and safety glasses when working on hazardous job sites.
- Devote your full attention to jobs that require heavy lifting. Often, accidents could have been prevented if the employee had been paying proper attention to the task at hand and lifting with their knees instead of their back. Always lift heavy items by bending your knees, and wear a back brace to prevent injury.

- If you need help, ask for it! Don't be embarrassed to ask for assistance with heavy lifting or if you don't understand completely how a task should be performed.
- Protect yourself against carpal tunnel syndrome.

For more information and tips about work safety, visit www. OSHA.gov.

30

Utilize Swimming Safety

There's more to it than just slapping on a pair of goggles!

Swimming is great exercise (excellent for toning) and very fun! You are weightless in the water and don't worry, your hair will survive. Enjoy swimming—just obey the rules!

Guidelines for safe swimming:
- Children should always be accompanied by an adult at the pool. Never leave children alone, even at home.
- Gates are around pools for a reason! Do not climb over gates or swim at public pools after hours when there isn't a lifeguard on duty.
- Always obey pool, beach, and lake rules. Read and obey all signage.
- Swim with a friend—two pairs of eyes are better than one!
- If you're just learning to swim, use a lifejacket or water wings. They aren't exactly cute, but they could save your life!
- Walk slowly in the pool area; never run.
- Only swim at depths you are comfortable with. If you are still learning to swim, stay in the shallow end where your feet can still touch the bottom.

- Do not push or jump on others. You could easily hurt some-one else or yourself.
- To avoid choking, don't chew gum or eat while you swim.
- If you suffer from seizures, or are with someone who does, be especially careful when swimming, and always notify the lifeguard and those around you of your condition.

Fact:

More than 25 percent of drowning victims are children fourteen and younger.

31

Know the Heimlich Maneuver

You never know when you might need it.

Did you know 60 percent of all choking victims treated in emergency rooms choked on food items, and 31 percent choked on nonfood items? (The other 9 percent are unknown or not recorded.)

Here is how to help save a choking victim:

- Reassure the victim that you know the Heimlich maneuver, and you are going to help them.
- If they are sitting, ask them to stand. If they can't stand, lift them up or ask others for assistance to get them standing.
- Position yourself behind the standing victim.
- Place your arms around their waist.
- Make a fist with one hand and place your thumb toward the victim, just above his or her belly button. Grab your fist with your other hand.
- Deliver five upward squeeze-thrusts into the abdomen. Each thrust will make the victim's diaphragm move air out of their lungs.
- Make each squeeze-thrust strong enough to dislodge a foreign body.

- Keep a firm grip on the victim.
- Repeat until the foreign object is expelled.

Avoid the risk of choking in the first place by chewing your food thoroughly, staying away from hard candy (especially children), and not talking with a mouth full of food! Eating slowly also helps digestion.

32

Know and Avoid Your Allergens

They're everywhere, just trying to make you miserable!

Be aware of your allergens and stay away from them when possible. To be safe, always check the label ingredients before you use a product. Educate those around you about the severity of your allergies and what to do if you experience a reaction. Wear a bracelet if you need to because allergic reactions can happen unexpectedly. Did you know that passionately kissing someone who has just eaten something you are allergic to can cause a severe allergic reaction? If you develop symptoms of an allergic reaction, seek medical attention immediately.

If you're not aware of any of your own specific allergens, take note of common allergens, such as latex. Some people can't even be around balloons because they have such a terrible allergy. Insect stings can also trigger allergies, the most com-mon allergens being bees, wasps, yellow jackets, hornets, and fire ants. Of course, not everyone is allergic to stings, but if you experience difficulty breathing, a rash that spreads beyond the area of the sting, swelling of the face, mouth, or throat, wheezing, anxiety, or rapid pulse, you might be experiencing a severe allergic reaction called anaphylactic shock and should get to an emergency room fast. Severe allergic reactions are not that common, but they can lead to shock, cardiac arrest, and unconsciousness in ten minutes or less. This type of reaction can occur within minutes after a sting and can be fatal.

Other common allergens are shellfish and nuts. If you are allergic to either of these things, avoid them at all times and be especially careful when dining out. If you have known allergies, carry an EpiPen whenever you can in case of a reaction.

Fact:

Peanut allergies are responsible for more deaths than any other type of allergy.

33

Try Strip Aerobics

Get down with your bad self.

When exercising is fun, you're a lot more likely to do it, right? I know that's how I feel! Running on a treadmill or lifting weights every day can get boring pretty quickly. If you're an adventurous spirit who likes to mix things up once in a while, try strip aerobics! These classes are high-energy, fun, and great for socializing with other ladies—not to mention releasing some of your inhibitions! You might even learn a few tricks that will really impress your husband or boyfriend.

If you're too shy to go alone, ask a few girlfriends to join you. There are even kits you can buy with a portable pole and DVD so you can have your very own class at home. Put on some fun music, turn the lights down, and start twirling! Just make sure the pole is properly secured—I don't want any of you ladies flying through a wall.

Some benefits of strip aerobics include interaction with others, flexibility (you've got to get down in those stilettos!), strength, balance, and endurance. It's fun!

So go ahead, ladies, give it a whirl!

34

Recognize the Signs of Depression

Sometimes it's more than just a bad day.

Depression is the most common mental health disorder in the United States among both teens and adults. About 20 percent of teens will experience depression before reaching adulthood. Depression varies from person to person, but there are some common signs and symptoms that you should be aware of. You may experience some or all of these symptoms as part of your normal life cycle. But keep in mind that the more symptoms you have, the more intense they are, and the longer they last, the more likely it is that you are suffering from depression.

It's time to seek help when these symptoms become overwhelming and interfere with your everyday life. If you become so depressed, you don't even want to get out of bed or get dressed in the morning, ask for help! Talk to your doctor about which symptoms you are dealing with in detail, and together you can find the best solution for you.

Signs of depression:
- Feelings of helplessness and/or hopelessness
- Loss of interest in daily activities
- Changes in appetite or weight

- Changes in sleep pattern and/or loss of energy
- Self-loathing
- Concentration problems
- Thoughts of suicide

For help and more information, visit www.psych.org.

Fact:

A regular vigorous exercise program can help keep depres-sion symptoms at bay.

35

Eat Whole Grains

An easy way to make your diet healthier!

Whole grains are a type of starch that is especially nutritious because they include the entire grain, which is comprised of the fiber, vitamins, and mineral-rich outer shell. Some studies show reduced risk of disease from as little as one serving of whole grains per day, though benefits are most apparent for those who consume at least three servings daily. The bottom line is that every whole grain in your diet helps—get them in there! Try incorporating whole wheat breads, pastas, and crackers into your meals as often as possible.

Benefits of eating whole grains:
- Better weight maintenance
- Reduced risk of asthma
- Lower risk of colorectal cancer
- Healthier blood pressure levels
- Less gum disease and tooth loss
- Reduction in risk of stroke and type 2 diabetes
- Reduction in heart disease risk by as much as 25–28 percent

So throw some oats in your next batch of cookies or on top of yogurt. Personally, I like to incorporate whole grains in every meal.

The U.S. Department of Agriculture's food pyramid recommends that adults eat at least three ounces of whole grains every day.

One ounce is approximately:
- I slice of whole-grain bread
- I cup of breakfast cereal
- ½ cup of cooked brown rice
- ½ cup of dry cereal
- ½ cup of whole-grain pasta

36

Know the Warning Signs for Alzheimer's Disease

Of all the things I miss, I miss my mind the most.

Alzheimer's, a progressive and fatal brain disease, is the most common form of dementia. Someone develops Alzheimer's every seventy seconds, and it is the fifth leading cause of death in the United States. It is more common in women, African-Americans, and some individuals with lower education levels. There is currently no cure for Alzheimer's, but treatments are available to control some of the symptoms such as agitation and aggression, and research to find a cure is ongoing.

A lot of my patients tell me their elderly parent or grandparent asks them the same question repeatedly or goes off to familiar places and then can't figure out where they are or how to get back home. If you experience situations like this with your loved ones, it may be time to have them tested. You should also speak with your doctor immediately if you notice symptoms like agitation or aggression in yourself or a loved one. Alzheimer's symptoms range from mild or moderate to severe.

The ten warning signs for Alzheimer's disease:
- Memory changes that affect daily life
- Challenges in planning or solving problems

- Difficulty performing simple tasks
- Confusion with time or place
- Trouble understanding visual images and/or spatial relationships
- New problems with words in speaking or writing
- Misplacing things and/or losing the ability to retrace steps
- Decreased or poor judgment
- Withdrawal from work or social activities
- Changes in mood and/or personality

You can help prevent Alzheimer's by keeping your body and mind exercised, controlling your diabetes and high blood pressure, and taking steps to prevent heart disease.

37

Keep Immunizations Current

Give it your best shot.

Don't hesitate, vaccinate! Vaccine-preventable diseases are at record lows. Even though most infants and toddlers have received all recommended vaccines by the age of two, many underimmunized children and adults remain, leaving the potential for outbreaks of disease—even diseases thought to be eradicated.

Adults, don't forget that there are vaccines for you, too! A live attenuated vaccine for shingles (Zostavax) received FDA approval in 2006 and is recommended for healthy adults sixty years of age and older. It may reduce the incidence of herpes zoster and PHN (postherpetic neuralgia). Isn't that amazing? Check with your doctor to see if you are a candidate for the shingles vaccination, an updated tetanus shot, the hepatitis series, the pneumonia shot, or the annual flu shot. Be sure to notify your doctor of any allergies you may have because allergens might be an ingredient in certain vaccines.

For the most current immunization information and schedules, visit the Centers for Disease Control and Prevention at www.cdc.gov.

38

Avoid Blood Clots and Deep Vein Thrombosis

Check your veins!

Deep vein thrombosis (DVT) refers to a blood clot that is usually embedded in one of the major deep veins of the lower legs, thighs, or pelvis. A clot blocks blood circulation through these veins, which carry blood from the lower body back to the heart. Symptoms occur in the affected leg when a clot obstructs blood flow and causes inflammation. Speak to your doctor immediately if you notice any of the following symptoms to keep the condition from worsening.

To prevent a blood clot, you should make sure to get up and stretch or walk on long flights, avoid sitting for extremely long periods of time, exercise, and eat healthy foods. And, of course, don't smoke! Varicose veins run in families, so know if you are at risk. Certain medicines have even been associated with clots, including hormones and birth control pills. You shouldn't smoke while taking these medications because it greatly increases your risk for developing a blood clot. When they go unchecked, blood clots can be fatal.

Symptoms of DVT may include the following:
- Swelling
- Gradual onset of pain

- Redness
- Skin that is warm to the touch
- Worsening leg pain when bending the foot
- Leg cramps, especially at night
- Bluish or whitish discoloration of skin

39

Know the Anatomy of a Label

Learn how to dissect food labels.

Before 1994, when the FDA and USDA begin regulating nutrition labels, food companies could print their products' nutrition information however they wanted, and it was often in very small print. Now that the information is readily available and easy to read, you should always look at the labels on foods you buy. Girl, you thought you were doing good with that energy drink, and you're actually drinking three and a half servings! One of the biggest things people fail to realize is that the first ingredient listed on the back of a product is what that product contains the largest quantity of. I can't tell you how many times I've bought "fat-free" or "reduced sugar" products only to flip them over and see that they are still mostly fat and sugar. Can you believe that? Here are the main things you should know about food labels:

The label indicates many things, including the percent-ages of vitamins, sodium, cholesterol, total fat, saturated fat, trans fat, protein, and total carbohydrates per serving. These are shown for a 2,000 (or sometimes 2,200) calorie per day diet.

Always check out the serving size, which is designed to reflect the amount an average adult would eat at one sitting. It's not always equal to the amount in the package.

Pay attention to saturated fat and cholesterol percentages. Both have been shown to raise serum cholesterol levels, which contribute to coronary artery disease. The American Heart Association recommends we limit our saturated fat intake to one-third of our total fat intake and cholesterol to less than 300 mg per day.

High fructose (refined sugar) consumption has been linked to heart disease and high blood pressure, cholesterol, and triglycerides—another type of fat that makes blood cells more prone to clotting. Try to limit your consumption.

You can avoid label reading altogether by shopping the perimeter of the market where the fresh fruit and vegetables are found. Sounds like a plan to me! Look out, lettuce and tomatoes, here I come!

40

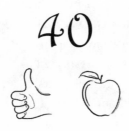

Fight Obesity

Put down the plate and step away from the buffet!

What three people are you eating for—me, myself, and I? Patients often come in and tell me, "Dr. Walker, I once was an ideal body weight. I was socially acceptable. Now, I look like a pumpkin with two legs!"

Obesity and being overweight pose a major risk for serious diet-related chronic diseases including type 2 diabetes, cardiovascular disease, hypertension, stroke, and certain forms of cancer. The health consequences of obesity range from increased risk of premature death to serious chronic conditions that reduce the overall quality of life.

Obesity has reached epidemic proportions globally, with more than one billion adults overweight, and at least three hundred million of these people clinically obese. It's not good to have it all hanging down, out, and about. Pot belly, chicken legs—oh, no! You are at a greater risk for heart disease if you are apple-shaped rather than pear-shaped. Obesity is a huge contributor to the global burden of chronic disease and disability. It is a complex condition with serious social and psychological aspects that affects all ages and socioeconomic groups. Child obesity is also a growing problem.

Increased consumption of more nutrient-poor foods with high levels of sugar and saturated fats, combined with reduced physical activity, has led to obesity rates that have risen nonstop since 1980. The obesity epidemic is not restricted to the United States either. In fact, this increase is often more drastic in developing countries.

So do something about it. Like I always tell my patients, "If it tastes good, spit it out!" Set a goal to remain at your ideal body weight, and keep your BMI (body mass index) within a normal range. If you are unsure about your BMI, calculate it using the formula below:

$$BMI = \text{Weight (lb)}/(\text{Height (in)} \times \text{Height (in)}) \times 703$$

41

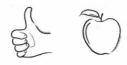

Prevent Food Poisoning

Is your tummy churning?

Food poisoning is no fun. Symptoms include abdominal cramping, nausea, vomiting, and an overall crappy feeling. Here are some precautions you can take to reduce the risk of food-borne disease:

Cook: Cook your meat, poultry, and eggs thoroughly. The biggest villains when it comes to food poisoning are fish, chicken, eggs, and mayonnaise. Check packages for cooking directions to make sure foods are cooked to the proper internal temperature.

Here are some rough guidelines:
- Fish and shellfish: 145 degrees Fahrenheit
- Beef, eggs, lamb, pork, and ham: 160 degrees
- Poultry: 165 degrees

Separate: Avoid cross-contaminating foods by washing hands, utensils, and cutting boards after they have been in contact with raw meat or poultry and before they touch another food.

Chill: Refrigerate leftovers promptly. Bacteria can grow quickly at room temperature, so refrigerate leftover food if it's not going to be eaten within four hours.

Clean: Always wash produce. Rinse fresh fruit and vegetables in running tap water to remove visible dirt and grime. Don't be a source of food-borne illness yourself. Wash your hands with soap and water before handling food, and use clean surfaces when preparing meals. You better not start cooking with a sink full of dirty dishes!

Report It: Report suspected food-borne illnesses to your local health department.

42

Prevent Strokes

Know how to help yourself avoid suffering from a stroke.

A stroke occurs when blood flow to your brain is blocked by either blood clots, narrowed blood vessels, or bleeding in the brain. Deprived of nutrients, the brain's nerve cells begin to die within a few minutes. As a result, a stroke can cause sensory and vision loss, problems with talking and walking, and/or difficulty thinking clearly. In many cases, the effects of a stroke are irreversible.

Did you know that approximately 800,000 people suffer from strokes each year? Or that women account for 60 percent of stroke related deaths? Or that strokes are the third leading cause of death in the United States?

Here are steps you can take to help prevent a stroke:
- Maintain a healthy blood pressure.
- Let your health-care provider know if you have a family or personal history of atrial fibrillation.
- Drink in moderation and don't smoke.
- Maintain healthy cholesterol levels.
- Take steps to keep diabetes under control.
- Exercise daily and eat a low-sodium diet.

Ask your health-care provider if you should get your homocysteine levels checked. Too much homocysteine in the blood may put you at greater risk for strokes, coronary heart disease, and peripheral vascular disease.

Ask your physician if any circulation problems you have could increase your risk of suffering a stroke.

If you experience any stroke symptoms such as sudden weakness of the face or a limb, blurred vision, dizziness, or an intense headache, seek immediate medical attention. Remember, time wasted is brain wasted.

Don't Underestimate the Importance of Pregnancy Health

You are not alone.

Being healthy throughout a pregnancy is extremely important for both the mom and the baby. Ideally, you should consult with your health-care provider and give yourself at least three months to prepare before trying to conceive. Pre-conception health means knowing how your health conditions and risk factors could affect you or your unborn baby. Being aware of certain health conditions that might affect your pregnancy (such as lupus, HIV, sickle-cell disease, herpes, or cancer) can help you make informed decisions regarding your pregnancy and health care. Also, talk to your doctor about what you can do to prepare your body.

Once you are pregnant, take care of yourself and your baby by:

- Getting early prenatal care: If you know you're pregnant or think you might be, call your doctor to schedule a visit. If you miss your appointment, reschedule. Make this a priority!
- Getting regular prenatal care: Your doctor will schedule you for many checkups over the course of your pregnancy. Don't miss any—they are all important.
- Following your doctor's advice.
- Eating healthy foods during your pregnancy: You should be doing this anyway, but it's especially important when carrying

your baby. Take all prenatal vitamins (such as folic acid) that your doctor prescribes.

- Asking questions: Knowledge is power. The more you know, the better you will be able to make smart, informed decisions for you and your child. There are hundreds of books on pregnancy and childbirth available to you. Most bookstores even have an entire section devoted to the topic. Do your research!

After giving birth, always be on guard and watch for symptoms of postpartum depression. Staying healthy during and after your pregnancy will ensure you are able to spend as much time with your child in this lifetime as possible.

Maintain Good Posture

Stand up straight!

Remember your mother telling you to sit up straight? Well, she was right. The spine has two natural curves called the double C curves, or the S curves, that you need to maintain. These are the curves found from the base of your head to your shoulders, and the curve from the upper back to the base of the spine. You should know the warning signs of back pain caused by poor ergonomics and bad posture.

Tips for improving your posture:
- Get up and move!
- Keep the body in alignment by standing straight up and making sure your weight is evenly distributed between both feet. Keep feet slightly apart, let your arms hang down naturally to the side of your body, and don't ever push your neck or chin out away from you.
- Keep your shoulders straight and aligned with the rest of your body.
- When you drive, sit with your back firmly against the seat.
- Be aware of posture and ergonomics at all times.
- Exercise to help prevent injury and promote good posture.

- Wear proper footwear at all times. Take a break from the stilettos once in a while, ladies! You look funny limping in them anyway. I wear mine every now and then, and when I do . . . oh baby, do I strut!
- Don't overdo it. Remember that it's important to maintain an overall relaxed posture. Clenching muscles and adopting an unnatural, stiff posture can ultimately restrict movement.
- S-t-r-e-t-c-h every morning, and be patient! It takes a long time to correct bad posture—even for you heavy-chested ladies when your chest is pulling you forward!

45

Stop Your Road Rage

Don't take your anger out on the road.

We all see drivers with road rage every day, but the cities considered to have the most drivers with road rage are Miami, Phoenix, New York, Los Angeles, and Boston. These are great cities. Come on, guys, let's turn it around! Chill out! In the olden days, people didn't even have the luxury of a car; they had to walk everywhere.

Several years ago, one of my patients witnessed a shooting, where a man who stopped at a railroad crossing was shot by the driver behind him for not speeding up and trying to beat the train. Isn't that crazy? Road rage should never escalate to this level. Here are some tips for stopping road rage in its tracks:

- Get enough sleep: We all know how easy it is to get cranky without enough sleep. It makes us prone to feelings of annoyance, resentment, and even anger. Eight hours or more is still the recommended daily amount of sleep for adults.
- Plan ahead: Plan your route in advance and give yourself plenty of time to get to your destination. Extra time equals calmer, more serene driving.
- Turn down the music: Listening to relaxing music rather than a driving bass line will make you less pumped up

for action. Try tuning in to a classical or jazz station to reduce stress, or listen to Zen music like I do!

- Breathe: Proper breathing reduces stress dramatically. Periodically roll down the window and breathe deeply and slowly.
- Be kind: Let other drivers go ahead of you. Slow down and let that jerk pass! Don't confront or follow someone who may have cut you off. If no accident or injuries occurred, let it go. Don't tailgate! Get back, Jack.

46

Breathe

It's more than waiting to exhale.

Most people seem to take breathing for granted. We just assume that it's something our body does naturally so we don't have to put much thought into it. Well, it may not require much thought, but putting a little into it is well worth the effort. Breathing is like a relationship—you're only going to get out of it as much as you put in.

Take a few minutes and try this exercise to become more aware of your breathing style. Start by closing your eyes and moving the air in and out of your lungs. Inhale through your nose and exhale through your mouth. Keep your back straight. Now start making an audible sigh when you exhale. Inhale as deep as you comfortably can, and then sigh as you push the breath out of you. Do this a few more times, and then continue without the sighing for at least eight or ten breaths. You should start to notice your body's optimum breathing rhythm. Open your eyes and continue breathing normally but with more awareness. This simple exercise can be done several times throughout the day to help calm your nerves and keep you relaxed by lowering blood pressure and your stress level. Don't shallow-breathe when you're feeling stressed—it won't help.

A good mental image I like to incorporate into my breathing exercises is imagining good things coming into my life when I inhale and bad things being pushed away when I exhale. This is very calming. If someone is stressing you out or things just don't seem to be going your way, take five minutes for yourself. Bring in the good with each breath, and exhale the negativity out and away.

47

Try Acupuncture

Needles aren't just for sewing and shots anymore.
Stick it to me!

Acupuncture is a painless alternative healing method that dates back to ancient Chinese times. It involves the insertion and manipulation of fine filiform needles into specific points on the body to relieve pain or fulfill other therapeutic purposes. The needles are typically left in place for about twenty minutes, though more acute and painful conditions usually require longer sessions. Acupuncture is usually given in courses of seven to ten daily treatments. After that, there's a break of several days before the next course begins. This schedule can be followed until the desired results are achieved. All you have to do is lie still! Many patients even fall asleep during treatment.

Acupuncture works directly with the body's energy, or *qi*. Practitioners believe the body becomes susceptible to illness when the natural flow of energy through the body becomes stuck, depleted, or weakened. Acupuncture promotes the body's rebalance through treatment of specific acupoints related to the symptoms or illness present. Treatment has been shown effective in removing these energy obstructions time and time again.

Acupuncture has been known to help treat:
- Respiratory disorders like sinusitis, the common cold, bronchitis, and asthma
- Toothaches
- Paralysis
- Osteoarthritis
- Chronic pain
- Infertility
- Anxiety and depression

Acupuncture is gaining a lot of momentum in the medical field. Visit www.acufinder.com to locate a licensed acupuncturist in your area.

48

Don't Text While Driving

Save the texting 'til you get home because what you've got to say isn't that serious.

Did you know that studies show the majority of people who believe text messaging while driving is dangerous do it anyway? About half of all adults who text, e-mail, or instant message from their cell phones admit to doing it while driving—even though they know they are endangering their lives and the lives of others. And more than one-third of all drivers under twenty-four admit to texting while driving. How much sense does that make?

In 2008, more than six thousand people were killed in automobile accidents involving a driver who was text messaging. So why are you sending a long, rambling text message on your phone about someone who did you wrong? You should be concentrating on the road! There's enough to concentrate on while driving without the added drama of phone calls and text messages.

It's been proven that if you text, e-mail, or instant message while driving, you are five times more likely to be in an automobile accident. Because of this, an increasing number of states now require drivers to use hands-free units while driving. It's not that easy, though. Early evidence shows there is also danger in hands-free phone use. This new information has prompted some states to prohibit using a telephone at all while behind the wheel. The safest thing to do is to always make your call upon arriving at your destination.

Simply talking on the phone reduces activity in the part of the brain responsible for driving by 37 percent. Experts say this is even worse for teenagers, who at most focus 50 percent of their attention on the road at any given time . . . so teenagers are in some serious trouble. The best rule of thumb? Keep your thumbs on the wheel, and talk and text only when you arrive at your destination.

49

Escape Stress-itis

Talk to the hand.

Over time, stress can have severe effects on your health. Consequently, learning how to avoid and reduce stress can help you live a longer, more comfortable life. Some health issues that can be caused or worsened by stress are high blood pressure, anxiety, depression, and difficulty sleeping. Think about what causes stress in your life, the nature of your stress response, and the negative effects you've noticed stress has on your body.

What are your main causes of stress? It could be your job, money, family problems, health problems, or many other things. Whatever they are, recognize them and deal with them. Here are some steps you can take for optimal stress management:

- Exercise! Because the stress response prepares us to fight or flee, our bodies are primed for action. So get to steppin' in that exercise class, girl! Exercise is a potent antidepressant, anxiolytic (meaning it combats anxiety), and sleep aid.
- Learn to laugh at yourself! I laugh at myself more than anyone. I'm funny, so why not?
- Stay away from toxic people. You know who they are! You were doing fine until you started talking to them on the phone, listening to them complain about how their life is messed up.

Just get them out of your life completely. Remember, people will never get tired of using you—*you* have got to get tired of people using you.

- Avoid alcohol and drugs; they only make matters worse. Try meditation, tai chi, Reiki, aromatherapy, or other relaxation techniques instead.
- Having sex (with your spouse) is also a great stress-reliever.
- Pray!

50

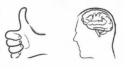

Prevent Headaches

What a pain!

Stress and tension are the top two causes of headaches. By learning to let go of the small things that irritate you, you are taking your first steps toward preventing future headaches. You've probably heard the old saying "Choose your battles," and it's very appropriate when it comes to headache prevention. If you have little or no control over a given stressful situation, teach yourself to roll with it. Make peace with the fact that nothing you can do will change the outcome, and learn to make the best of these types of situations. This is a valuable lesson for all areas of life!

Rolling with the punches isn't enough to prevent everyone's headaches. When it's not, managing your diet is another way to get your headaches under control. Many foods will aggravate or even trigger a headache, so be aware of what you eat.

Foods and drinks that can trigger a headache include caffeine, red wine, aged cheese, chocolate, eggs, alcohol, fatty foods, and fast food.

Try avoiding these foods and eating a small salad or drinking warm apple juice, cider, or water with lemon instead. Staying well-hydrated also greatly reduces your chances of getting a headache. So save yourself some misery, girl, and relax! Make the most of your

131 years by having as few headaches as possible. This should also help make phrases like "You are about to make me blow my stack!" obsolete.

51

Try Meditation

Find your own mantra.

Having trouble relaxing? Meditation is an excellent ancient method for calming the body, mind, and spirit. Sometimes it seems impossible to find a little quiet time in our hectic lives, but taking as little as five or ten minutes a day to sit in a relaxed, upright position, take a few deep breaths, and concentrate on tranquil thoughts can make a world of difference in your mental health. Just don't fall asleep! Meditation can also help lower your blood pressure, elevate your mood, and calm your nerves.

If you have kids, tell them you will be unavailable for ten minutes each night and that they are not to disturb you. Remember, you've got to take care of yourself before you'll be any good to anyone else. You know what they say, when Mom's not happy, nobody's happy. Ain't that the truth?

There are hundreds of CDs available with music that is suitable for meditation. New age and metaphysical stores are a great place to look. Some of my favorite CDs are those that feature nature sounds like rain falling, ocean waves, or the rainforest. Try a few and find one that puts you at ease. I like to have Zen music playing softly while I do my meditations. Try some aromatherapy for an added benefit. My favorite scents for meditation are eucalyptus and jasmine. So relaxing!

"Let my soul calm itself, O Christ, in thee."
—H.B. Stowe

"He restores my soul."
—Psalm 23:3

52

Listen to Music

*Music calms the savage beast that lurks so
close to the surface in all of us!*

Did you know that music has the power to soothe, calm, and heal you?
If you love Mary J. Blige like I do, you know this is true! The idea of
using music as a healing method is hundreds (maybe even thousands)
of years old. The twentieth century version of this discipline began
after World War I when both amateur and professional musicians
went to hospitals to play for the thousands of veterans who were
suffering from physical and emotional trauma. The patients' notable
physical and emotional responses to the music led doctors to request
that their hospitals hire the musicians. Today, we have music therapists
who are trained and licensed to use rhythm, tone, and notes to help
their patients. Music therapy is now commonly used in hospices and
home health-care services all over the world.

Music has been shown to affect portions of the brain that relate
to mood, emotions, and social interactions. New benefits are being
discovered all the time, but currently, therapists are seeing that music
can lift your spirits, counteract depression, promote movement for
physical rehabilitation, calm, sedate, counteract fear, and lessen
muscle tension. For instance, research suggests that listening to
Mozart's Piano Sonata K448 can reduce the number of seizures in
people with epilepsy. This is referred to as the "Mozart Effect."

Music is used to help children, adolescents, adults, and the elderly, as well as patients with mental health problems, learning disabilities, Alzheimer's disease, substance abuse problems, brain injuries, physical disabilities, and chronic pain. Ask your health-care provider if music therapy might be beneficial for you.

To find a music therapist in your area, visit the American Music Therapy Association website at www.musictherapy.org.

53

Practice Tai Chi

Slow it down and act like a warrior.

Tai chi (sometimes called tai chi chuan) is a noncompetitive, self-paced system of gentle physical exercise and stretching. In tai chi, you perform a series of postures or movements in a slow, graceful manner. Each posture flows into the next without pausing. Anyone, regardless of age or physical ability, can practice tai chi because it doesn't take much physical prowess. Instead, tai chi emphasizes technique over strength.

Tai chi is used to:
- Reduce stress
- Increase flexibility
- Improve muscle strength and definition
- Increase energy, stamina, and agility
- Increase feelings of well-being

Tai chi has more than one hundred movements and positions. You can find several that you like and stick with those or explore the full range. The intensity and pace of tai chi varies somewhat depending on the form or style practiced. However, most forms are gentle and suitable for everyone. I have a patient who attends a tai chi class designed just for seniors with arthritis. Some of these motions can even be performed while talking on the phone or performing other household chores. Talk about multitasking! Tai chi can help you reduce stress and increase your quality of life through relaxation, mental focus, and light physical activity.

54

Try Aromatherapy to Relax

The power of smell can heal.

Aromatherapy is the practice of using plant oils for psycho-logical and physical well-being. Essential oils (the pure essence of a plant) have been found to provide both psychological and physical benefits when used correctly and safely. I feel so good when I go to Bath & Body Works or Pier 1 Imports to stock up on fragrant soaps, oils, and candles. My home is truly an aromatic oasis!

When inhaled, essential oils offer both psychological and physical benefits. (It's important to note that these oils should never be applied to the skin in their undiluted form.) These oils can enhance your mood, trigger pleasant memories, and calm your nerves. In addition to therapeutic benefits, essential oils are helpful in other applications. They can be used in household and laundry cleaners, and some oils act as a natural insect repellent and pesticide. You may recall using citronella candles during the summer to keep mosquitoes away. Citronella oil is the ingredient in the candles that is responsible for repelling the mosquitoes.

Essential oils can also be mixed together to create appealing and complex aromas that can be used for specific therapeutic application. Aromatherapy practitioners can custom blend a scent just for you. Some of my favorite scents for relaxing are lilac, lavender, eucalyptus, and spearmint. A diva always keeps herself and her home smelling fabulous! I rub a little on at bedtime after using my eucalyptus sugar scrub in the bath, and I sleep so well. So go out and get some good scents up in here! Up in here!

55

Check for Breast Cancer

Don't be shy—know your breasts!

One in eight women will develop breast cancer in her lifetime. I am dedicated to keeping you informed about early detection.

Breast cancer is the seventh leading cause of death in the United States. In 2008, 186,467 women and 1,764 men were diagnosed with the disease. There are a couple of things that you should do regularly to check for breast cancer in the early stages. First, know the possible signs of breast cancer and watch for them:
- Pain in the breast or surrounding area
- Skin thickening around the nipple and/or inverted nipple
- Breast lumps
- Nipple and/or breast discharge
- Change in breast size, shape, or texture

Some of my patients also report a severe itch in the breast area when cancer is involved.

You should perform a self breast exam (SBE) every month to check for any of these signs. Do this at least one week after your period, or you're likely to feel a little bit of everything in there! Finally, know when to get a mammogram and do it. A mammogram is an X-ray of your breast that detects tumors, even those that cannot be felt during an SBE, as well as tiny deposits of calcium that may indicate the presence of breast cancer.

There are two types of mammograms: routine and diagnostic. Women forty and older should have a routine mammogram every one to two years. If you are at a higher than average risk of breast cancer due to a family or personal history of cancer, you may need a mammogram more often. Check with your health-care provider about the best screening schedule for you. You should have a diagnostic mammogram if you notice anything unusual in your SBE or exhibit any of the signs of breast cancer.

Visit www.komen.org for more information.

56

Know about Menopause

Menopause means mustache. Sorry, ladies, but it's true!

The definition of menopause is menses pause, hence the name, menopause. Menopause is the transition period in your life (late forties for most women) when your ovaries stop producing eggs, your body produces less estrogen and progesterone, and menstruation becomes less frequent before eventually stopping altogether. When the estrogen production in your ovaries starts to decline, androgen production increases, and you get a mustache. Oh, ladies . . . I hate to bust you out like that! Common symptoms of menopause in women include:

- Racing heartbeat
- Craving sweets (ice cream appears to be your vice of choice)
- Weight gain
- Hot flashes and skin flushing
- Depression, irritability, and anxiety (sometimes with no identifiable cause)
- Insomnia and night sweats
- Sometimes—a funky attitude

Now to relieve some of those menopause symptoms, let's try taking that exercise program up a notch! When extra exercise isn't enough, treatment with hormones may be helpful for severe symptoms such as hot flashes, night sweats, or vaginal dryness. Discuss the decision to take hormones thoroughly with your doctor, and weigh your risks against any possible benefits. Pay careful attention to the many options available to you that do not involve taking hormones, such as soy products and homeopathic remedies (for example, try drinking cool water with celery stalks for hot flashes!). Every woman is different. Your doctor should be aware of your entire medical history when considering prescribing hormone therapy. And remember, the shorter the therapy, the better.

57

Know about Male Menopause

Divorcing your wife of thirty-five years to marry your eighteen-year-old girlfriend in a feverish attempt to resurrect your youth? Play on, player!

Are you over fifty and getting that spare tire around your waist? Do you feel tired a lot? Not as sharp as you used to be? Experiencing less drive and ambition? Muscles sore? You may be experiencing signs of male menopause. That's right, men, there is such a thing after all! Did you know that if you're overweight, your body can have lower than normal levels of testosterone, and it can actually convert some of your testosterone into estrogen? Yes, I said it! Some of you men can have a little more estrogen onboard than others. Even if you're not overweight, there is a gradual decline in testosterone as men age, and it isn't just your sex drive and libido that suffer. Other systems in your body such as your brain, nervous system, muscles, and circulatory system are also impacted by testosterone.

And you've been wondering why the old gray mare ain't what she used to be. You hit the bedroom, you're willing, but you just aren't able! But there is help. After age forty, ask your doctor if you need to have your testosterone levels checked. I can just see you guys walking in there with your head hanging low, asking your doctor, "Isn't it about time for a baseline testosterone level check?" In the meantime, here are some ways to help prevent symptoms of male menopause:

- Stay active.
- Lose weight.
- Eat more broccoli, brussels sprouts, cabbage, and cauliflower, and load up on as many leafy green vegetables as possible!

Some studies have shown that zinc, vitamin C, vitamin E, and supplements that are rich in antioxidants can also help with symptoms.

Exercise and eat up!

58

Eat More Fruits and Vegetables

Bugs Bunny had it right all along!

A diet rich in fruits and vegetables has been shown to reduce the risk of certain cancersand other chronic illnesses such as high blood pressure, heart disease, and even Alzheimer's. It can also contribute to improved digestive health and improved joint health. To reap these benefits, I recommend you eat five to nine servings of fruits and vegetables each day.

A serving is considered one medium-sized piece of fruit or vegetable (about a quarter of a cup) or four ounces of juice. And by all means, eat a variety because that's the best way to get the beneficial antioxidants, fiber, minerals, and vitamins your body needs. You'll get a great boost of energy this way. You're going to look good and feel even better. One easy way to increase your servings is to try some dried fruit as a tasty snack. You can take it anywhere! On the run, I like to drop a prune or two. But please be mindful of the sugar and carbohydrate content, which can be high.

Vegetables come in an array of wild colors and flavors. Down south, my grandmother affectionately called turnip greens the bitter greens because of their bitter taste. Vegetables are loaded with antioxidants, fiber, vitamins, minerals, and phytochemicals.

In the next couple of chapters, I'll tell you how to pick and store fruits and vegetables. For instance, ripe tomatoes are completely red or reddish orange. They have a sweet aroma and yield slightly to gentle palm pressure. When I was growing up, we simply walked out the back door, picked a fresh tomato, and ate it.

Sweet potatoes should not be refrigerated. Store them in your pantry or another cool, damp place. Look for sweet potatoes that are thick and tapered toward the ends. You can store them with an apple to keep them from sprouting. I love sweet potato ice cream. Check out my website for a delicious recipe!

Shop for compact, firm, and green brussels sprouts. Fresh sprouts should be kept in your refrigerator and can be steamed, simmered in water, or sautéed until tender. Try serving them with 2 percent shredded cheese. Give these sometimes underappreciated vegetables a try! And don't say you don't like it until you've tried it!

59

Know How to Pick and Store Fruit

Get a passion for fruit.

Cantaloupe: Smell the stem! If it has a sweet aroma, it's ready to eat. To keep it fresh, seal in an airtight container in your refrigerator. Serve some delicious wedges for breakfast.

Apples: You want your apples to have a vibrant, bright color. They should be firm to the touch, not mushy or easily imprinted by your thumb. For optimum freshness, apples should be stored in the refrigerator.

Grapes: Choose grapes that are plump, smooth, and evenly colored. Store in a plastic bag in the refrigerator, and be sure to wash them before serving.

Oranges: Look for oranges that have a fresh appearance and feel heavy for their size. To keep them fresh, store in a plastic bag in the refrigerator or in the crisper. They taste delicious chilled! Valencia oranges also make good juice, so go for it, girl! Make some homemade orange juice for your boo. Squeeze it!

Pears: Don't be so rough! You ain't squeezing on a man! Pears have to be handled gently. To ripen a pear, place it in a brown bag at room temperature. Once they're ripe, store unwashed pears in the refrigerator. Try serving with low-fat cottage cheese.

Pineapples: Look for dark green leaves and a fresh, bright appearance. Serve fresh in salads or grilled on a kabob with purple and white onions and cherry tomatoes. What a colorful treat next to some grilled salmon. Mmm!

Peaches: Peaches are best eaten as soon as they are ripe. I love fresh peaches on top of soy pancakes. And they're from Georgia just like me! That's right, I am an official Georgia Peach. Don't be jealous!

Bananas: I never met a banana I didn't like. Bananas should be smooth and evenly colored, not bumpy, lumpy, or bruised.

60

Know How to Pick
and Store Vegetables

Popeye knew what he was talking about.

Greens: Select greens with fresh, crisp leaves, and try to pick the darkest, greenest color you can find. They should be cleaned and stored in the crisper section of your refrigerator. The rule of thumb for greens in general is to rinse them off with water that has a little salt in it to get rid of soil and other things that have a tendency to stick to the leaves. I like to combine different greens and sauté them in a little olive oil and garlic as a side dish.

Lettuce: Choose the nutritious, darker green varieties. Lettuce can be stored in the crisper in your refrigerator. Mix several different types together for a delicious salad. I like to layer it on a plate with some fresh fruit on top. Yum!

Cauliflower: Choose a heavy, firm cauliflower with minimal discoloration. Keep it dry and refrigerate in a plastic bag. Serve with low-fat dressing for a tasty snack.

Broccoli: Choose broccoli with purplish or green heads—never yellow. Store unwashed in the refrigerator and serve with low-fat cheese or in a salad.

Cabbage: Choose a heavy and compact head of cabbage that has no discoloration. Use in a coleslaw or stir-fry. Red cabbage jazzes up fresh salads quite nicely! My favorite is steamed cabbage with a little olive oil.

Asparagus (so misunderstood!): Choose bright green stalks that are straight with closed tips. Slender spears are usually more tender. Store in the coldest part of your refrigerator with the base wrapped in a damp towel.

Carrots (the eyes have it!): Select carrots that are bright orange, firm, and free of dark spots or blemishes. I enjoy a glass of carrot juice every morning. You should try it!

61

Eat More Berries

They're berry nice!

If you've ever had the pleasure of picking ripe berries from a garden or gathering wild berries in the woods like I have, you already know how wonderful they are. Most berries are naturally sweet and require little effort to prepare. Just rinse them under water and serve for a nutritious snack or dessert.

Cranberries (not just for Thanksgiving anymore!) are powerful antioxidants that help prevent tooth decay and urinary tract infections. Trying using them in a low-fat vinaigrette.

Raspberries are a good source of vitamin C and manganese. They have less sugar than most fruit and are highly nutritious as well. They make an excellent snack!

Strawberries are a great source of vitamin C. They are nutrient-dense and fabulous alone or in a healthy smoothie, sugar-free ice cream, or a delicious spring salad.

Blueberries are a food with one of the highest concentrations of antioxidants. They also have a moderately low amount of sugar compared to other fruit, and are a good source of vitamin C, vitamin K, and manganese. There is also some evidence of reduced cancer and heart disease risk from eating blueberries. I know Martha Stewart can give us a fabulous recipe for blueberries!

Blackberries are a very good source of vitamin C, manganese, and vitamin K. They are delicious alone or in smoothies, sugar-free pies, and sugar-free jams.

I love all berries and incorporate them into my diet almost daily. They're easy to prepare, delicious, and great for your health. My best recipe: rinse them off and eat them! Find out what berries are native to your state and take your children berry-picking!

62

Acai Berry

What a wonderfully powerful antioxidant!

The acai berry, relative of the blueberry, cranberry, and other dark purple fruit, is an inch-long reddish-purple fruit. Acai berries come from the acai palm tree, which is native to Central and South America. Research on the acai berry has focused on its powerful antioxidant qualities. Theoretically, it may help prevent diseases caused by oxidative stress such as heart disease and certain cancers. To understand oxidation, think of slicing an apple in half. Over time, the inside of the fruit turns brown. Our bodies are not so different. Oxidizing processes in the body make normal cells turn abnormal, just like the flesh of the apple turning brown.

Acai contains two substances called anthocyanins and flavonoids. Anthocyanins, named for two Greek words meaning "plant" and "blue," are responsible for the red, purple, and blue hues in many fruits, vegetables, and flowers. Foods and drinks that are richest in anthocyanins (blueberries, red grapes, red wine, and acai) are very richly colored, ranging from dark purple to black. Anthocyanins and flavonoids are extremely powerful antioxidants that help defend your body against life's stressors. They also play a role in cell protection. Eating a diet rich in antioxidants may inhibit the aging process and help prevent disease by neutralizing free radicals, which are harmful byproducts produced by the body. Talk about a win-win situation!

While the full benefits of acai are still unknown, the antioxidant properties it possesses are reason enough to give it a try. Of course, fresh acai berries are the best way to reap the benefits of this magical fruit, but unfortunately they are not readily available to most of us. The next best thing is to find a reputable company that produces acai in supplement form. Incorporating acai into your diet may be a good choice for you, but, as always, speak with your health-care provider before taking any supplements.

63

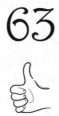

Stop Nuclear War

Can't we all just get along?

Disarm. Enough said.

Let us not forget the courageous men and women who have protected our freedom. Veterans Day is November 11.

64

Take Charge of Your Finances

Unless you're rolling serious paper like Jay-Z, have the business mind of Craig Jerabeck, or possess the financial wizardry of Suze Orman, you need to be ballin' on a budget!

The last time I can recall not being in debt was when I was in the third grade. Why are you laughing? Don't play dumb; you know that's you, too! Living within your means can be difficult—especially when you make very little and have a mailbox full of past-due bills waiting for you every night when you get home from work. But it can be done; don't get discouraged! Most creditors are willing to work with you. If you can, try to live below your means, not above them. Here are ten steps to help you take charge of your finances:

- Check your credit reports once a year (it's free) and correct any errors you may find.
- Make a monthly budget and stick to it.
- Set aside a little each month for a rainy day.
- Pay more than the minimum payment on your credit cards.
- Take only the money you can afford to spend when you go shopping.
- Don't apply for any more credit cards. Girl, you can't pay your Visa with your MasterCard!
- Pay off the credit cards with the highest interest rate first.
- Don't lend money to friends or family unless you can afford to not be repaid. Refer them to an FDIC-insured bank instead.

- Start a three-month emergency fund that will cover your bills.
- Skip expensive dinners and make meals at home. A peanut butter and jelly sandwich and some vegetable soup sounds good to me . . . I eat it all the time!

The Credit Bureaus:

Experian: 1-888-397-3742
Equifax: 1-800-685-1111
TransUnion: 1-800-888-4213

Remember, your health is your wealth.

65

Consider a CoQ10 supplement

Revitalize your cells.

Organs such as the heart and liver have the highest energy require-ments and the highest CoQ10 concentrations.

Coenzyme Q10 (or CoQ10) is naturally produced by your body and is necessary for your cells to function normally. Unfortunately, your body's CoQ10 levels decrease with age. Patients with heart disease, Parkinson's disease, cancer, diabetes, HIV/AIDS, or other chronic illnesses are also more likely to have lower than normal levels. These levels can be increased by taking a CoQ10 supplement. CoQ10 is still a little controversial, and some of its benefits are still unknown, but I have patients who swear it has lessened their pain substantially.

Studies have shown CoQ10 to be beneficial in the treat-ment of:

- Hypertension: People with high blood pressure have often been found to have low levels of naturally occurring CoQ10 in their bodies.
- Alzheimer's disease: Studies have shown CoQ10 might help to slow down (but not cure) dementia in individuals with Alzheimer's.
- Angina: If you suffer from clogged arteries, CoQ10 may help improve your body's ability to tolerate rigorous exercise.

- Migraines.
- Kidney failure.

New studies are taking place all the time, and I'm sure we'll be hearing a lot more about CoQ10 in the next few years. Until then, if the information you've read here has sparked your interest, talk to your health-care provider and find out if a CoQ10 supplement is right for you.

66

Eat More Honey

It's nature's nectar . . . and it can help you lose weight!

For over four thousand years, honey has been used for everything from calming a simple cough to helping with weight loss. Ancient Egyptians sacrificed honey by the ton to their river gods. The Romans slathered honey on battle injuries to reap benefits from its antibacterial qualities. It was used as a sweetener for foods until the use of refined sugar from sugar cane became the norm. Even now, there are many things honey can do for us.

Because of its considerable carbohydrate content, honey is a great energy booster. Try consuming one or two tablespoons for an extra boost before you head to the gym for a few miles on the treadmill. Honey also has natural antioxidant qualities that are great for helping your digestive system run smoothly. It's commonly used as an ingredient in effective home remedies for treating small cuts and burns, yeast infections, athlete's foot, and some arthritis pain. It's also great for sore throats, hangovers (don't tell anybody I gave you a hangover remedy!), and sleeplessness (milk and honey).

Did I mention how absolutely delicious honey is with other foods? My all-time favorite honey "recipe" has to be a little organic honey drizzled on top of a banana. Oh! My mouth is watering just thinking about it. I might even risk smudging my lipstick for one of those bad boys! Oh my goodness . . . honey is just plain fabulous and a wonderful way to ensure you live 131 years filled with sticky and sweet goodness.

Facts:

- Honey supplies energy at sixty-four calories per table-spoon, which fuels your working muscles.
- Its lubricating qualities make honey a good gentle laxative.
- A mixture of honey and ginger is an excellent expectorant and may provide relief to a person suffering from cough, cold, sore throat, and/or runny nose.

67

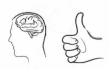

Dress for Success

When you look good, you are more likely to succeed.

If you are poorly groomed with spots all over yourself, bad breath, messy hair, cheese butt, and clothes that are three sizes too small, you are setting yourself up for a really bad day. Looking good is an essential part of feeling good, and feeling good is an essential part of being successful at work and in life.

Think about how your clothes make you feel. Do they emphasize your good features? Or do they hug you in all the wrong places and make you feel insecure and unsure of yourself? My dad used to tell me that, even when he had little or no money, he still put on his best clothes and went out into the world to seek out opportunities. His handsome appearance gave him the confidence he needed to make a better life for himself, and I am proud to say he accomplished a lot in his lifetime. They say clothes make the man. Well, I say they make the woman, too. In fact, a woman probably picked that man's outfit out anyway, so ladies, it really is up to us!

Dress for success daily checklist:
- Does this outfit make me feel confident?
- Are these colors flattering to my skin tone?
- Is what I'm wearing appropriate for the weather?

- Am I dressed appropriately for where I'm going? Is it a formal or informal event?
- Are these shoes too small?
- Can I comfortably wear this outfit for several hours?
- Does what I'm wearing restrict my movement in any way?
- Are all my tags concealed?
- Am I bulging at the seams? Can you see my Spanx?
- Do I look like a hoochie Barbie?

Being successful contributes to a longer and healthier life. I love getting dressed every morning, and so should you! What woman doesn't enjoy clothes? The world is my runway, darling. When I wear burgundy scrubs to the office, you can bet my lipstick matches!

68

Buy Some Apple Cider Vinegar

The apple elixir!

Hippocrates (the father of modern medicine) was known to use vinegar mixed with honey as an energizing tonic and a healing elixir.

Apple cider vinegar is made from the fermentation of apple juice to hard apple cider, followed by a second fermentation that yields the apple cider vinegar. Organic apple cider vinegar retains all the nutritional goodness of the apples from which it was made, plus it's supercharged with the extra acids and enzymes that are produced during fermentation. It's easily found in most grocery stores and can be used for weight loss, acne, warts, bruises, burns, cuts, and constipation. Plus, it's completely natural—which you know I love!

Apple cider vinegar contains acetic acid and small amounts of malic acid, lactic acid, and various other amino acids. These acids give it antiseptic properties that help prevent the growth of unwanted bacteria and yeast in your digestive tract. Taking a little apple cider vinegar before a meal can increase stomach acidity and improve digestion and nutrient absorption. It also contains pectin, a water-soluble fiber that can absorb fat, toxins, and cholesterol in the digestive tract and remove them from your body. Good-bye and good riddance! It has a host of easily absorbable minerals too, with potassium being the most plentiful. Potassium works together with sodium to control the body's water balance, conduction of nerve impulses, contraction of muscles, maintenance of normal heart rhythm, and your body's storage and breaking down of carbohydrates for energy.

Keep in mind: all bottles of apple cider vinegar are not created equally. Use the kind made from cold pressed, organically grown apples. This means no chemicals or preservatives have been added, and it is not pasteurized. Try taking one tablespoon of apple cider vinegar and one tablespoon of honey in a glass of warm water twice a day to help lower blood pressure. I take a whopping teaspoon every morning as I head out the door—mmm! This is not for the faint of heart though; vinegar has an intense flavor and aroma, so be prepared!

69

Cook with Olive Oil

You Italian stallion!

Olive oil is a natural juice that preserves the taste, aroma, vitamins, and properties of the olive fruit. It is native to Italy and Greece where the olives are crushed to release the oil inside. It takes a lot of olives to make some olive oil! There is about one tablespoon of olive oil in:

- twenty medium Mission olives
- forty small, ripe black olives
- twenty jumbo, ripe black olives
- seven super colossal, ripe black olives

The resulting oil is a triglyceride, meaning it is made up of three fatty acids attached to a glycerol backbone. Triglycerides are the major energy reserve for both plants and animals. The beneficial health effects of olive oil come from its high content of both monounsaturated fatty acids and antioxidants. Studies show that people who eat antioxidant-rich foods, such as olive oil, vegetable oil, fruits, vegetables, grains, and nuts, have a lower chance of getting heart disease and cancer. It can help protect against heart disease by controlling LDL (bad) cholesterol levels, while raising HDL (good) cholesterol levels. No other naturally produced oil has as large an amount of monounsaturated fatty acids as olive oil.

Olive oil is also very well tolerated by the stomach. In fact, its protective function has a beneficial effect on ulcers and gastritis. It also activates the secretion of bile and pancreatic hormones much more naturally than prescribed drugs. Consequently, olive oil lowers the incidence of gallstone formation. Incorporating olive oil into your cooking and diet is definitely not a bad idea!

I love to stir-fry fresh veggies in olive oil and serve them atop a bed of whole-grain pasta. It's absolutely delicious! Want some?

70

Eat Ginger

An exciting and unusual natural remedy.

Ginger has been used as a natural remedy for centuries in island cultures and Asia. Now science is catching up and researchers around the world are finding that ginger works wonders for treating everything from cancer to migraines. Ginger is extremely popular in the Caribbean islands, where it grows wild. Jamaica, known for the strong flavor of its ginger, currently provides most of the world's supply, followed by India, Africa, and China.

Potential health benefits of ginger:
- Colon cancer prevention
- Morning sickness remedy
- Motion sickness remedy
- Reduction of pain and inflammation
- Heartburn relief
- Cold and flu prevention and treatment
- Migraine relief
- Menstrual cramp relief
- Prevention of diabetic nephropathy

Ginger is available in six forms: fresh, dried, pickled, preserved, candied, and powdered/ground. The root is the most potent part of the plant. Ginger is peppery and sweet, with a pungent aroma. Keep in mind that fresh ginger turns bitter if you burn it, so be careful when cooking. Ginger can be included in sauces or seasonings and is great with sushi or a salad. Personally, I love gingersnaps! They taste great and are low in sugar, so they make an excellent snack if you're watching your sugar levels.

71

Use More Cinnamon

A delicious way to improve your health.

Cinnamon has a long and fabulous history. Centuries ago, this incredible spice was used for embalming and preserving meat. Medieval physicians used cinnamon in medicines to treat coughing, hoarseness, and sore throats. Cinnamon has been used as currency and even has aphrodisiacal qualities. Hey now!

Did you know that just half a teaspoon of cinnamon per day can lower LDL cholesterol? Several studies suggest that cinnamon may have a regulatory effect on blood sugar also, making it especially beneficial for people with type 2 diabetes. This magical spice has even shown an amazing ability to stop medication-resistant yeast infections. Hard to believe, isn't it? And most of us have a bottle sitting right in our spice rack!

Cinnamon also has an anticlotting effect on the blood. In a study at Copenhagen University, patients given half a teaspoon of cinnamon powder with one tablespoon of honey every morning before breakfast had significant relief of arthritis pain after one week and could walk without pain within one month! When added to food, cinnamon inhibits bacterial growth and food spoilage, making it a natural food preservative. One study found that smelling cinnamon boosts cognitive function and memory. It has even been shown to help fight E. coli bacteria in juices that are not pasteurized.

Try incorporating cinnamon without sugar into your diet and witness a little bit of this healing magic for yourself! But don't go telling people I told you to go out and eat a whole pan of cinnamon rolls. I did not say that!

72

Try Cod Liver Oil

Grandma's cure-all remedy.

When my siblings and I were young and didn't feel good, my grandma would line us all up and give us each a whopping dose of cod liver oil. And you know what? We felt better! In a study conducted at Cardiff University in Wales, people with severe osteoarthritis who took cod liver oil capsules for twelve weeks showed a considerable reduction in enzymes that cause damage to cartilage and joint pain. These researchers have proven what Grandma said all along! They hailed it as a breakthrough in arthritis treatment and a way to reduce the rising demand for joint replacement operations.

Osteoarthritis, the breakdown of the cartilage that cushions the joints, causes pain and stiffness in millions of people as they grow older. Cod liver oil is believed to decrease inflammation, so people with rheumatoid arthritis (an inflammatory disease) often take fish oil supplements to help reduce symptoms. Hey, anything's worth a try if it is natural, legal, and can lessen your pain. If you have arthritis, ask your health-care provider if you should try cod liver oil to see if it helps. Even if it turns out that fish oil doesn't help your arthritis, there are other known benefits it can provide.

Reported benefits and uses for cod liver oil:

- It's high in vitamins A and D, which is helpful because most adults don't get the recommended daily allowance of vitamin D.
- It improves the appearance of hair, skin, and nails. Maybe you can eventually break away from those wigs and acrylic nails, ladies, and we can stop being a "weave of nations"!
- It can also be used on small burns to prevent blistering. Remember, serious burns should always be evaluated by a doctor.
- It may aid in improved brain and heart function.

You can find cod liver oil almost anywhere! Try your local health food store, supermarket, or neighborhood pharmacy. I just run around the corner to my neighborhood Schnuck's.

73

Consider Trying Biofeedback

The mind-body connection.

Biofeedback is a type of alternative medicine called mind-body therapy that's designed to enable you to use your thoughts and will to control your body. It's based on the idea (confirmed by scientific studies) that people have the ability to influence many of the automatic, involuntary functions of their bodies with their minds—and I agree! Biofeedback has helped me conquer my terrible migraine headaches.

Biofeedback can be particularly useful in treating stress-related conditions, anxiety, and depression. Clinical trials are evaluating its benefits in the treatment of many other conditions including asthma, headaches, hot flashes, Raynaud's disease, irritable bowel syndrome, nausea and vomiting associated with chemotherapy, irregular heartbeats (cardiac arrhythmias), chronic low back pain, and chronic constipation.

Sessions are performed by a therapist who specializes in biofeedback. Preparation depends on the type of therapy used, but typically sessions last from half an hour to an hour. The length and number of sessions is determined by your condition and how quickly you learn to control your physical responses. During your session, a therapist will apply electrical sensors to different parts of your body. These sensors will monitor your body's physiological response to stress. When you begin to recognize that your pain is a result of tense muscles, the next step is for you to learn how to invoke positive physical changes in your body, such as tightening and relaxing specific muscles when your body is physically or mentally stressed.

Get More Antioxidants

They're leading the fight against free radicals.

Antioxidants mostly find their way into your body through the foods you eat. Once inside, they can slow down or even prevent the oxidation of other molecules. Recall my example from an earlier chapter where I compared oxidation in the human body to an apple cut in half. The exposed inside of the apple turns brown due to oxidation. When molecules in your body oxidize, they can create free radicals, which are organic molecules responsible for aging, tissue damage, and some diseases. These molecules are very unstable, and therefore they look to bond with other molecules, destroying their good qualities and perpetuating the bad ones. Antioxidants, present in many foods, are molecules that prevent free radicals from harming healthy tissue. It is normal to have these free radicals in your body, but an excessive amount is bad for your cellular structures.

The most effective way to expose yourself to more anti-oxidants is through your diet. By incorporating at least five to nine servings of fruits and vegetables a day into your diet, you may be helping your body reduce its chances of heart disease, neurological diseases, cancer, and lowered immunity—just to name a few benefits. Examples of common antioxidants include glutathione, beta-carotene, vitamin C, vitamin A, selenium, alpha lipoic acid, melatonin, and vitamin E.

Foods that have strong antioxidant properties:

- Blueberries, cranberries, blackberries, and strawberries
- Prunes
- Pinto beans, red beans, and kidney beans
- Apples, carrots, broccoli, cauliflower, greens, and spinach
- Russet potatoes (Eat the skin! You'll also get some potassium, fiber, and vitamin C.)

75

Clean Up Your House

Cleanliness is next to godliness.

A clean home or work environment truly is the key to being your most productive. It's hard to be productive in a house full of crap, isn't it? First of all, you can't find anything in all that clutter. Second, how are you going to concentrate on your work knowing there are germs crawling all over the place? I can't stand working in unclean conditions. It just makes me feel dirty. Pass the bleach and Pine-Sol! Before you relax for an evening at home or start a project at work or school, take five or ten minutes to wipe down surfaces with antibacterial wipes, sweep or vacuum dirt and debris from the floor, and clean those mirrors and windows. You'll be amazed at what a difference this can make. And make sure you get all your dirty clothes off the floor, put them in a laundry basket, wash them, fold them, and put them away. Don't leave them in the basket for weeks at a time. Dust your surfaces! Get rid of that pet dander! And by the way, dust mites are real bugs. Just know that when you're in bed sleeping at night, they are looking at you. . . .

Tips for a clean home:
- Declutter: wear it, give it away, or trash it.
- Sweep your kitchen floor and wash your dirty dishes daily. I

am not eating at your house if I peep in your kitchen and see two weeks of dirty dishes piled up. No thanks!
- Clean up messes when they are fresh. Dried liquids are much more difficult to remove.
- Clean your bathroom two to three times per week. Germs live there!
- Vacuum carpets and mop wood floors weekly.
- Wash windows and mirrors frequently.
- Use air freshener or scented candles to keep your space smelling wonderful. Open windows occasionally to let in fresh air.

Clean up, clean up, everybody do their share!

76

Learn to Deal with Your Dysfunctional Family

Is your family missing the "function"
part of dysfunction?

When circumstances such as parental alcoholism and/or drug addiction, hostile divorce, mental illness, child abuse, or extremely controlling parents interfere with a family's ability to function, the children can be affected long after they have grown up and left their problematic families.

Family dysfunction can be any condition that interferes with healthy family interactions. Most families have periods of time where their bonds are impaired by stressful circumstances (a death in the family, a parent's serious illness, etc.). However, healthy families tend to get back to functioning normally after they've worked through the crisis. In dysfunctional families, problems tend to be chronic, and children oftentimes do not get their basic needs met.

I say it's time to break the generational curses, pick yourself up, dust yourself off, and make a decision to move on. The most painful things in the world are our secrets.

Steps to help you move on:
- Practice taking care of yourself and your needs first. When I fly Delta, they always say, in case of an emergency, "Put the mask on you first." This is good advice for all areas of your life.

151

- Allow yourself to feel angry about what happened, and then let it go and move on.
- Talk about your feelings with a counselor, therapist, or your pastor.
- Begin to change your relationship with your family by keeping an open line of communication.
- Try to sit down and eat dinner with your family nightly.
- Stay spiritually grounded. Wear life like loose-fitting clothing.

77

Get a Pet

*I don't care if it's 100 percent purebred
or 100 percent mutt.*

Did you know that the unconditional love of a pet may help lower your blood pressure, triglycerides, and cholesterol levels? The comforting effect pets have on their owners may help lower blood pressure and stress levels, which in turn may promote protection from heart disease. Pet owners who suffer heart attacks are also more likely to survive than non-pet owners. Studies conducted on people with AIDS and senior citizens indicate that pet ownership can also help significantly relieve symptoms of depression.

Pets also seem to meet the need for companionship and relationship building that is not available to some people. Senior citizens who own pets are better able to tolerate social isolation and are more active than those who do not. Activity levels were actually higher in those with pets, regardless of the kind of pet the individuals owned. For many, the sense of responsibility associated with caring for a pet is significant. Nurturing an animal may even increase a person's ability to form friendships with people.

If you are financially able to provide for a pet, you might consider getting one to help improve your mood and contribute to a long and happy life! Man's best friend might help you heal. My first pet was a beautiful little white dog named Snowball. Currently, I own goldfish because I'm not home enough to care for a dog. My fish are so peaceful, so calm.

If you decide to get a pet, be prepared for pet ownership. Remember, you should always spay or neuter your pet, and animals get sick just like people. Take into consideration vet bills, food, leashes and collars, training, and pet-sitting if you're away for long periods of time. And don't forget to clean up after your pet—I better see you out there with the pooper scooper!

Someone may be waiting to give you some love!

For more information, visit the ASPCA website at www.ASPCA.org.

78

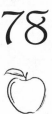

Bake, Broil, and Grill

Say good-bye to the French fry!

There are many ways you can turn grilling into a healthy way to eat and also a fun and flavorful way to cook. By choosing foods that are low in fat, high in nutrients, and full of flavor, you can prepare tasty meals that are also good for you. Marinades are great because they not only add extra flavor, but they also reduce the formation of cancer-causing substances on foods. A marinade containing olive oil and/or citrus juices can reduce the formation of these chemicals by as much as 99 percent while also helping to tenderize the meat. For a healthier option, try using herbs and spices instead of sauces and marinades that can be full of fat, calories, and sugar.

There has been a lot of talk about grilling and cancer, so make sure you don't burn your food when you grill. The risk is real, and you need to keep it in mind, but don't worry, there are simple things you can do to reduce it. For those of you who are interested, the two primary substances that form on over-grilled food and could cause cancer are heterocyclic amines (HCA) and polycyclic aromatic hydrocarbons (PAH). Simply put, these chemicals are formed by putting food (primarily meat) in contact with intense heat and flame. HCA and PAH are known cancer-causing agents, so you need to reduce their formation as much as you can by not overcooking or burning meat on the grill. And please don't add grease to meats you're about to broil or bake—most meats make their own. You don't need a double dose of grease! Come on, now. . . .

Cooking should be fun and delicious, but it doesn't have to be fattening! Cooking healthy is something I do every day. One of my quick and easy recipes is sautéing some broccoli, spinach, and sliced cherry tomatoes in a skillet with just a little olive oil and a little low-fat shredded cheese. Add three egg whites (yes, I said three; I'm a healthy girl!) and scramble together. Serve with one slice of whole wheat toast. Yum!

79

Prepare for the Unexpected

Expect the best but prepare for the worst.

Does your family have a plan in case of an earthquake? What about a tornado, a fire, or even a terrorist attack? Do you know who you would call in case of emergency? Are their phone numbers handy? Being prepared for these kinds of disasters can save lives and help you remain calm during times of crisis.

Tips for staying prepared in all areas of your life:
- As a family, discuss what you should do in case of a tornado, hurricane, fire, flood, or terrorist attack.
- Purchase a weather radio for use during storms.
- Keep flashlights and plenty of batteries in your home and car.
- Have an extra supply of water and nonperishable food where it is easily accessible.
- Keep a list of emergency numbers on your refrigerator and in your nightstand. Make sure all family members know where the list is and who to call for what.
- Program all local hospital numbers into your cell phone.
- Know the best route to local hospitals and trauma centers.
- Install a security alarm.

- Use antivirus and identity theft protection software on all home computers.
- Talk to your children! Educate them about sex, drugs, and what to do when a stranger approaches them on the street. Knowledge is power—you can trust me on that.

80

Stop Addictions: They're Equal Opportunity Destroyers

The best way to quit is never to start.

Addictions are compulsions to use and abuse things like drugs and alcohol to an excessive and destructive extent. These powerful compulsions can produce a self-perpetuating, life-threatening process that can end in disability or death for the sufferer and cause family members and loved ones pain and suffering. Additionally, addictions can create medical problems and cause poor dental hygiene, dry skin, thinning hair, bad breath, and an unkempt appearance.

You can help young people avoid addictive drugs like alcohol, marijuana, cocaine, heroin, amphetamines like crystal meth, sleeping pills, tranquilizers, and pain medications. The best things to do are:

- Live by example; hang out with drug-free people.
- Talk to your kids early about drugs; the pushers do!
- Make sure they're getting drug education at home and in school.
- Never accept any unknown substance from anyone.

There are thousands of emergency room visits each year due to illegal drug use. Marijuana is the most commonly used illicit drug in the United States, with 6 percent of children twelve years and older admitting to use within the previous month. The rate of illicit drug use is highest among those eighteen to twenty years of age. In my practice, I'm seeing a lot of old men trying crack for the first time. You know you're too old to be a space cadet!

If you have an addiction, get help by contacting a medical professional who specializes in addictions. Ask your health-care provider for a referral to an inpatient or outpatient rehab facility, or contact your local Alcoholics Anonymous or Narcotics Anonymous chapter. You've got to want to help yourself first.

81

Keep Yourself Safe from Murders and Homicides

Make personal safety your number one priority at all times.

Homicide refers to both criminal and noncriminal (justifiable) murder. Criminal homicide means killing someone intentionally, during the commission of another crime, or due to recklessness, emotional outburst, or provocation. In the United States, murder charges require intent or malice aforethought, which also includes transferred intent (when a criminal's intent to harm one person accidentally results in harm to a second person).

According to the FBI's Child Abduction and Serial Killer Unit, child abduction and serial homicide are the most serious violent crimes in the United States. Homicide is the second leading cause of death for people fifteen to twenty-four years of age and the leading cause of death for African-Americans and Hispanics in the same age group. For every violent death, there are one hundred nonfatal injuries caused by violence. We've got to put an end to this!

How you can prevent murders and homicides:
- Make sure children don't have access to firearms by keeping them locked up. Keep ammunition in a separate place where it can be locked up too.
- Enroll children in after-school programs.

- Lock your doors, and never open the door to a stranger.
- Be aware of your surroundings at all times.
- Stay in well-lit areas.
- Try to exude confidence at all times. Predators often seek out individuals who appear vulnerable and less confident in public.
- Get out of relationships that are physically and/or verbally abusive. Get a restraining order if necessary, and report all violations immediately.
- Be leery of people who are looking to take out large insurance policies on you—especially if they are broke.

Fact:

In 2008, New Orleans had the highest murder rate of any city in the United States. Come on, y'all! You don't have anything better to do?

82

Don't Tolerate Domestic Violence

There's no excuse for an abusive relationship.

One in three women will be a victim of domestic violence in her lifetime.

Did you know that approximately 1.3 million women and 835,000 men are physically assaulted by an intimate partner in the United States every year? I can remember working in the emergency room as a junior medical student and seeing my first case of domestic violence. This patient's husband had beaten her left eye out of its socket and rendered it useless. In her case, love was literally blind.

Some signs of domestic abuse include always wearing dark glasses, extreme insecurity or very low self-esteem, constantly making excuses for their spouse, social isolation, and acting fearful of their spouse or scared of upsetting them. If someone had offered this patient help earlier, maybe this incident wouldn't have happened. Watch for these common signs of domestic violence in your friends and family members.

Domestic violence and abuse are used for one purpose only: to gain and maintain total control of a relationship. An abuser doesn't play fair. Abusers use fear, guilt, shame, and intimidation to wear down their victims and keep them under their thumbs. Abusers may also threaten their victims, hurt them, or hurt those close to them. Domestic violence and abuse does not discriminate. It happens among heterosexual couples and in same-sex partnerships. It occurs to people of all ages, ethnic backgrounds, and financial levels. Though women are more commonly victimized, men are also abused—especially verbally and emotionally.

Domestic abuse often escalates from threats and verbal abuse to physical violence and sometimes even murder. While physical violence may be the most obvious danger, the emotional and psychological consequences of domestic abuse are sometimes just as harmful. Domestic violence hurts more than just the primary victim. The negative impact on children who witness domestic violence is immeasurable. If you or someone you know is a victim of domestic violence, I want you to know that there is help available to you. You shouldn't have to live in fear anymore. No one deserves to live like that. Your first step toward breaking free is recognizing that your situation is abusive. Once you acknowledge the reality of the abusive situation, then you can get the help you need. Don't ever let anyone slap you around!

If you've got to quit me, please don't kill me.

For more information about domestic violence initiatives, visit www.avonfoundation.org.

83

Learn How to Deal with Infidelity

Grits: they're not just for breakfast anymore.

This is a touchy subject for many, but I'm including it here because I feel that to live a long and fabulous life, you really need to know this information. Think of how many people get shot in the butt, sliced with a knife, mowed over, or have acid or hot grits thrown in their face by their spouse because they were unfaithful.

Infidelity is any time you go outside of your marriage or committed relationship for a sexual encounter of the third kind.

One of the worst cases of infidelity that I know of involved a married man who lived a double life. No one knew he had been unfaithful to his wife for thirty-two years until he died of a massive heart attack. His wife found out that he had also fathered children with his mistress when the mistress and her children (who showed a striking resemblance to her late husband and her children) showed up at the funeral.

When we have been cheated on, many of us begin to lie to ourselves to try to get through the difficult time. I'm here to give it to you straight. When you have been betrayed, there is so much going on sometimes that we don't know what to think. You may feel lonely, insecure, depressed, and inadequate or be plagued by worry, self-doubt, and trust issues. Here are the two things I want you to remember when it comes to infidelity:

- It is not your fault.
- Chances are that it will happen again.

Although we may never know the exact number of cheaters out there because affairs are clothed in secrecy and hidden agendas, estimates have infidelity occurring in at least 25–50 percent of all marriages. Even though infidelity is most common in men, y'all women are cheating, too! Don't play! It's also most common in people under thirty, people with a history of multiple sexual partners, and people who have to spend a long time away from their spouses, like traveling salesmen.

What you do is up to you, but please remember these two truths. I wouldn't lie to you. Make the decision that is best for you because this is one time in your life when you've got to put yourself first and trust God. To recover from infidelity, start by taking life one day at a time, and take time to remind yourself of the positive things in your life. Don't dwell on the past or keep bringing it up in conversation with friends or family. Keep yourself healthy and moving forward. Exercise daily and don't revert to junk food for comfort—it will only make matters worse!

Fool me once, shame on you. Fool me twice, shame on me. We won't even get into unwanted pregnancies and the spread of STDs. Spare me the baby-mama drama! Remember this story in the Bible—King David desired Bathsheba, who was married, and had her husband, Uriah, killed so he could have her for himself. . . .

Practice Gun Safety

There's no kidding around when it comes to firearms.

Approximately five hundred children are accidentally killed in the United States each year because they were playing with a gun at home or at a friend's home.

- Use a firearm safe or lock box in conjunction with a trigger or chamber lock when storing firearms.
- Store and lock ammunition in a separate place.
- Remove firearms from your home if you have a depressed or suicidal family member.
- Before you send your child to someone's house, ask if firearms in the home are stored unloaded and locked. Ask if the ammunition is stored separately. Be sure to check on shotguns and rifles, too, not just handguns.
- If you have doubts about the safety of someone else's home, invite their children to play at your home instead.
- Talk with your children about the risk of firearm injury in places they may visit or play.
- Teach your child to know that if he or she finds a firearm, they should leave it alone and let an adult know right away.
- Never play with guns—they are not toys. And they are certainly not for Russian roulette. Don't even playfully point

a gun at someone who may not know if it's real or not—
especially the PoPo!

The United States is the leader in gun deaths among industrial
nations, which has resulted in various gun control laws at the federal
and state levels. It doesn't matter if you're for or against guns, you
should understand gun safety rules and teach them to your children.
Accidental gun deaths are totally preventable. I encourage you to
take the steps necessary to ensure you and your loved ones are never
harmed by a gun in your home (or anywhere). Burglars beware: when
you break in a house, you're likely to get blown up!

85

Battle Fears and Phobias

What are you afraid of?

Fears and phobias are not uncommon, but for some people they are crippling, sometimes even leaving them housebound. When this happens, it's time to do something about it.

Some common fears are: fear of disease, sickness, or poor health, fear of dying, fear of airplanes and flying, fear of failure, fear of public speaking, fear of small spaces, and fear of animals, bugs, and/or spiders.

There is help, though. Through a combination of behavioral techniques and cognitive therapy, you can overcome your crippling fears and phobias. Behavioral treatments usually consist of relaxation, desensitization, and sometimes medication. Cognitive therapy involves direct exposure to the feared object or situation.

Here are some of my favorite tips for battling fear:

- First, confront your fears. The first step is to identify your fear and quit trying to run from it. Confront the problem head-on, and make a plan that consists of small steps you can take to gradually overcome your fear. For instance, someone who is afraid to fly might start by first getting on a stationary plane.

- Try using positive motivation. Try not to dwell on the negative things. Knowing what you can do is much better than focusing on what you can't.
- Try to see failure and rejection in a new light. Often it's easier to not do something because we fear failure and rejection. For example, you may fear failure when starting on a new career path. Or maybe you fear rejection by friends, family, and the people around you if you fail. Just stay positive and focus on all the good things that can come of making a change. Remember, a failure or rejection is just another opportunity waiting to be taken.

86

Get Plenty of Sunshine

Here comes the sun!

Twenty minutes of sunshine each day can improve serotonin production in your body, which in turn improves your mood.

Yes, sunshine is a good thing when taken in moderation. Vitamin D, which helps us grow and maintain strong, healthy bones, is produced by your skin in response to exposure to ultraviolet radiation from natural sunlight. Some research even suggests that vitamin D may provide protection from some diseases and conditions such as cancer and hypertension. Exposure to sunshine is even more important for obese people—they need twice as much vitamin D because their bodies don't utilize it properly. Twenty minutes of sunshine a day is all it takes to help prevent several conditions:

- Osteoporosis, which is commonly caused by a lack of vitamin D
- Rickets, a bone-wasting disease
- Seasonal affective disorder, which is caused by a melatonin imbalance initiated by lack of exposure to the sun

Exposure to the sun and healthy vitamin D levels can even help relieve symptoms of depression.

Chronic vitamin D deficiency is often misdiagnosed as fibro-myalgia because its symptoms (muscular weakness, aches, and pains) are so similar. If you're exhibiting symptoms like these, you should ask your health-care provider to see if you need your vita-min D levels checked. In the meantime, go out for an early morn-ing walk and enjoy the sunshine. Don't forget your sunscreen and sunglasses! And remember, avoid direct sun exposure between 11 a.m. and 3 p.m.

You are my sunshine, my only sunshine. You make me happy!

87

Don't Drive Drunk

Just don't do it.

On average, someone is killed by a drunk driver every forty-five minutes.

Did you know that over 1.46 million drivers were arrested in 2008 for driving under the influence of alcohol or narcotics? This is an arrest rate of one for every 139 licensed drivers in the United States. So why are you out there driving drunk, acting like a fool? Somebody grab the keys, please!

Every single injury and death caused by drunk driving is totally preventable. Although the number of crashes that are alcohol related has dropped in recent years, there are still far too many. Unfortunately, in spite of great progress, alcohol-impaired driving remains a serious national problem that tragically claims thousands of victims annually. Drivers with a blood alcohol content (BAC) that is higher than .15 are frequently involved in accidents that result in death. In 2008, an estimated 11,773 people died in crashes where the driver had a BAC over the legal limit of .08.

So know your limits (usually about two drinks) and drink responsibly. The best rule is, if you're going to drink, have a designated driver. Or skip the drinking altogether and have a bottled water or spritzer instead! Don't risk drinking and driving. It's not worth risking your life, the lives of others, having your license suspended, or having a device put on your car that requires you to breathe into it before the car will start!

For more information, visit the Mothers Against Drunk Driving website at www.MADD.org.

Don't Speed

You don't need to get anywhere that fast.

Approximately 41,500 people lose their lives in the United States each year in a speeding-related accident. Slow down and save lives.

Speeding is one of those things I just don't understand. I find it hilarious that someone will rev their engine and speed past me, only to meet me again at the stoplight just up the road. Hello, it's me again! It just doesn't make sense. Why not leave home a little early so you can take time getting to your destination? It's so rare for me to have alone time that I treasure my little road trips so I can be in the car alone with my good thoughts. What could be better than me time?

Unfortunately, it's apparent that not everyone feels the same way because speeding-related fatalities are on the rise on roads with a speed limit of 65 mph or more. Men are most likely to be involved in a speeding-related crash, and most of these accidents occur on weekends. Many speeding-related deaths also involve drugs and/or alcohol. Nearly half of all alcohol- or drug-impaired drivers exceeded the speed limit before fatal crashes, compared with 14 percent for sober drivers. Here are a few tips on how to slow down:

- Just slow down, period!
- Leave home five or ten minutes earlier, and allow yourself more time to travel to your destination.

- Plan your route in advance to avoid getting lost and having to make up time.
- Don't talk on the phone, eat, or drink while driving. Studies show avoiding distractions can help you stay focused on driving the speed limit and greatly reduce the risk of accidents.
- Put down the makeup, diva.

I want to dedicate this chapter to all the policemen, firemen, and road workers who are keeping our streets and highways safe and in great condition. You guys rock! A lot of you are cute, too! Watch out for those drivers who are texting or driving with their music blasting. They don't hear you or see you.

89

Start a Garden

The most natural way to stay grounded. Literally!

Gardening is an excellent hobby because it's inexpensive, fun, and relaxing. Sure you'll get a little dirty, but you'll have fun doing it, and feel a sense of accomplishment when your seeds grow into beautiful fruits, vegetables, and other plants. There's something very satisfying about putting your hands in the dirt and connecting with the Earth. There are many other benefits, too:

- It gives you a feeling of accomplishment.
- It may reduce stress.
- It burns calories!
- You can save money by planting your own veggies.
- You can grow herbs and spices to cook with—yum!
- Kids love to get involved and help out. As an added bonus, they will usually eat what they grow.

What you need to get started:

- Raised flower boxes for above-ground gardening
- Gloves
- Annuals and perennials
- Shovels
- Pots

- Watering can
- Fertilizer
- A willing attitude

Don't wanna go outside? Bring the plants inside and grow herbs and spices in your windowsill!

90

Take a Belly-Dancing Class

I know some of your bellies dance every time you walk,
but that's not what I mean. I'm talking exercise!

The origins of belly dancing, though not totally clear, can be traced to the Middle East, the Mediterranean, and Africa. In times past, belly dancers were highly sought after because belly dancing was considered much more extravagant and mystical than local dances.

It's also another fun way to get some exercise outside of a gym. Have you seen those girls shake? Now that takes talent! They aren't just entertaining the crowd; they're burning calories, too! You can't beat that. And belly dancing is not a thin woman's dance, believe me.

While belly dancing might not be for everyone, it's worth a try if you're bored with traditional exercise. Many women also find that belly dancing helps them feel more connected to their bodies and more in touch with their sexuality. Hey, whatever works! When attending a class, you should wear something comfortable and loose-fitting that is easy to move in. There is no need to wear a belly-baring shirt to class unless you want to. If you want to get into it, you can wear a hip scarf, finger cymbals, and any other belly-dancing gear you own, but this is not required. So go ahead, shake that belly! And if you can't find a belly-dancing class near you, go to a toy store and grab a Hula-hoop! Roll it, girl!

Remember how tiny Jeannie's waist was?

91

Educate Yourself about
Drug Interactions

*It's important that you understand the possible
consequences of mixing drugs.*

A drug interaction occurs when the effect of a particular drug
is altered when taken with another drug or with food.

Drugs are foreign chemicals to the human body that are
digested just like the food we eat. When a drug is taken orally,
it usually travels from the stomach to the liver, where it is
metabolized (this is the process of breaking down and removing
chemicals from the body). As the drugs pass through the liver or
small intestine, the cytochrome P450 family of enzymes breaks
them down.

If drugs interact with the wrong thing, this process can be
altered, and in some cases the results are harmful. There are
three kinds of drug interactions: drug/drug (i.e., atorvastatin
and ketoconazole), drug/food (i.e., fluvoxamine and grapefruit
juice), and drug/disease (i.e., prednisone and diabetes). Mixing
two drugs together or mixing a drug with the wrong food could
make the drugs ineffective. The combination can also increase a
drug's effect, which may be harmful. The result might be mild
symptoms such as nausea, stomach upset, or headache, or more
serious problems such as a dramatic drop in blood pressure,
irregular heartbeat, or damage to the liver.

To avoid harmful effects, you should never, under any circumstances, take a medication that is not prescribed for you. You should also avoid alcohol when taking prescription medications and know if your medicine should be taken with or without food. And always keep your doctor in the loop. It is important to talk with your physician or pharmacist when starting or stopping a drug to prevent harmful interactions and to get the best therapeutic outcome. You should also make sure your health-care provider is aware before you switch to generic medications.

92

Protect the Rainforest

We can't let such a valuable resource be destroyed!

Did you know the world's largest pharmacy is not on your neighborhood corner after all? It's actually the rainforest, which is known for the large number of natural medicines discovered there.

Rainforests are forests that are characterized by heavy rainfall— on average 68–70 inches annually. Tropical rainforests can be found in the tropics and areas such as South America and Southeast Asia. There are temperate rainforests in more moderate regions of the world such as North America, Ireland, and southern China.

A tropical rainforest is typically divided into four main layers. The emergent layer contains a small number of very large trees and is populated by wildlife like eagles and monkeys. Next is the canopy layer, which contains most of the larger trees. The next layer, called the understory layer, is home to a number of birds, snakes, lizards, and predators such as jaguars and leopards. Insect life is also abundant here. The bottom layer, called the forest floor, receives only about 2 percent of sunlight. Because only plants adapted to low-light conditions can survive here, many forms of fungus grow on the forest floor where they help decay the animal and plant waste.

Did you know that 40–75 percent of all species on Earth are indigenous to the rainforest? Or that the rainforest provides us with timber, meat, and plant-derived medicines? Rainforests are top tourist destinations and extremely beneficial to the ecosystem as a whole. However, some species of plants and animals are being driven to extinction by rapid deforestation. Preserving the numerous exotic animal and plant species found in the rainforest is extremely important for not only the overall health of the planet but also for medical research. It's important that we all do our part to help save the rainforest. One good way to help is to get involved with the Rainforest Foundation, which was founded by that good-looking Sting and his wife, Trudie Styler, in 1989.

For information on how you can help save the rainforest, visit www.rainforestfoundation.org.

93

Eat a Low-Fat Diet

A low-fat diet equals a low-fat you!

Eating a low-fat diet has many health benefits, including reducing your risk of stroke and heart disease, while helping you to maintain a healthy weight. Below are some of my favorite tips for low-fat cooking and dining:

- Trim all visible fat from beef and poultry, and remove the skin from poultry before eating.
- Bake, broil, or roast meat dishes instead of deep-fat frying them. To prevent drying and add flavor, baste with wine, lemon juice, or low-fat broth.
- Try experimenting with herbs and spices such as dill, tarragon, cilantro, and basil. They jazz up otherwise ordinary meals.
- Use black pepper to add flavor. I love black pepper on everything. I even blacken my grits!
- Avoid fatty sauces and gravies.
- Minimize your use of butter.
- Minimize your use of products, such as margarines, that contain partially hydrogenated oils—this limits trans-fats.
- If pan- or stir-frying, use small amounts of vegetable oils such as canola or safflower oil. You should also increase your use of olive oil.

- Cut down on whole-milk products by switching to 2 percent or 1 percent milk. If you want to be really good, try transitioning to skim milk.
- Stay away from those crab leg specials! Shellfish is loaded with cholesterol.
- Drink a lot of water! Add lemon wedges to make it more flavorful.
- Limit fried foods. I see a lot of people eating fried desserts nowadays, and I hope this is one trend that passes. You don't need a fried candy bar! We've taken fried food to a whole new level of misunderstanding.

94

Eat a High-Fiber Diet

It keeps things running smoothly.

A high-fiber diet (20–30 grams per day for both men and women) offers many health benefits, from reducing your risk for colon cancer to keeping common digestive disorders at bay. If you're not used to eating a lot of fiber, take it easy at first or you may experience gas, diarrhea, bloating, or abdominal pain. You should also increase water intake to make it easier on your digestive system. To fully transition to a high-fiber diet, you should:

- Start slow by adding a little fiber to your diet each day until you reach around 30 grams per day. This gradual progression will allow the bacteria that are found naturally in your digestive system to adjust to the high-fiber diet.
- Drink half your body weight (in ounces) of water each day (unless you have a health condition that requires you to limit your fluid intake).
- Try a supplement if you have specific dietary restrictions that prevent you from altering your diet.

There are two types of fiber, soluble and insoluble, both of which are undigested. This means they are not absorbed into your bloodstream. Instead of being absorbed and used for energy, fiber is excreted from your body. Insoluble fiber passes through our intestines largely intact. To increase your daily intake, try some of these foods—they're all high in fiber:

- Whole-grain and whole wheat products such as bagels, bran, brown rice, buds, cereal, granola, muffins, and pasta
- Dried fruit (apricots, dates, prunes, raisins), apples, avocados, bananas, blackberries, blueberries, mangos, oranges, peaches, pears, raspberries, and strawberries
- Vegetables such as broccoli, carrots, cauliflower, corn, green beans, green peas, greens, and potatoes
- Beans like black, garbanzo (chick pea), kidney, lentils, lima, pinto, and soy

95

Get a Stress Test

"Wherever you go, go with all your heart."
—Confucius

Some heart problems are easier to diagnose when your heart is working hard and beating fast. This is where stress testing comes in—it gives your doctor information about how your heart works when it is under physical stress. During a stress test, you exercise on a treadmill or bicycle to make your heart work hard and beat fast. While you exercise, your doctor will perform different tests on your heart. The whole test usually takes less than two hours, is not painful, and requires no anesthesia.

Doctors typically use stress testing to help diagnose coronary heart disease (CHD), also called coronary artery disease. CHD is a condition in which a fatty material (plaque) builds up in your coronary arteries and narrows the arteries, which reduces blood flow to your heart. It also makes it more likely that blood clots will form. Blood clots are dangerous because they can partially or completely block the flow of blood through your heart, which can lead to chest pain or a heart attack.

You might need a stress test if you have a family history of heart disease, abnormal EKGs during a routine physical, chest pain/angina, diabetes, or if you've recently recovered from a heart attack or heart surgery. Any young person with a family history of heart disease should be evaluated. If you've already been diagnosed with CHD, a stress test may also be performed to see how severe your condition is. This can help extend and improve the quality of your life by helping your doctor determine what kind of treatment you need.

Ladies, if you think only men need to be concerned about heart attacks, you're wrong. Ten years after you start menopause, your chances of suffering a heart attack are equal to a man's—even if you have no family history of heart disease. Be proactive and get a stress test.

"A cheerful heart is good medicine."
—*Proverbs 17:22*

"Do not let your hearts be troubled."
—*John 14:1*

96

Wear a Helmet

It's a requirement, not a fashion statement.

Did you know that on average, 85–90 percent of the seven hundred cyclists who die each year were not wearing a helmet when they crashed? Or that 540,000 bicyclists visit emergency rooms with injuries every year? Of those, about 67,000 have head injuries, and 27,000 have injuries severe enough that they are hospitalized. So what can you do to protect your head, skull, and brain while you're riding a bike or participating in a dangerous job or sport? Wear a helmet!

The oldest known use of helmets dates to about 900 BC when Assyrian soldiers wore thick leather or bronze helmets to protect them during battle. Today, helmets are used for recreational activities and sports, for dangerous jobs such as construction, and while traveling on a motorcycle or bicycle. Even Barbie wears a helmet when she rides her pink bike! How do I know? Because I've got one just like it! Helmets save lives and prevent head-crushing injuries. Head trauma is a common cause of childhood hospitalization, so please, educate your children about the importance of wearing helmets.

Other tips for helmet safety:

- Buy yourself and your kids fashionable helmets in a color you like—you all will be more likely to wear them if you like them.
- Always make sure your helmet fits properly. The shell and pads should be firm and sturdy, and the straps should be snug.
- Choose a helmet with proper ventilation.
- Wear a helmet at all times when cycling, skateboarding, roller skating, or rollerblading—even if the state doesn't require it.
- Remember that a helmet and good cycling skills go hand in hand. Even though you're wearing a helmet, it's still important to always practice safe riding.

Get a Prostate Cancer Screening

It could save your life—it's as simple as that.

Cancer is a group of abnormal cells that grow more rapidly than normal cells and refuse to die. Prostate cancer is one of the most common types of cancer, affecting about one in six men in the United States. The prostate is a small, walnut-shaped gland in males that produces seminal fluid. Prostate cancer usually grows slowly and initially remains confined to the prostate gland. If prostate cancer is detected early—when it is still confined to the prostate gland—you have a better chance of successful treatment.

Some men exhibit no symptoms of prostate cancer. For most men, prostate cancer is detected during a routine screening such as a prostate-specific antigen (PSA) test or a digital rectal exam (DRE). However, some men show symptoms like trouble urinating, decreased force in the stream of urine, blood in the urine, blood in the semen, swelling in the legs, discomfort in the pelvic area, bone pain that doesn't go away, bone fractures, and/or compression of the spine. If you notice any of these symptoms, talk to your doctor right away.

You are at higher risk for prostate cancer if you are over fifty, have a family history of prostate cancer, eat a high-fat diet, and/or have high testosterone levels. For reasons that aren't well understood, African-American men also have a higher risk of developing and dying of prostate cancer. So remember, get regular checkups (especially after age fifty), eat a healthy diet, and keep up your screenings. Although effective treatment is available with early detection, prevention is always better.

98

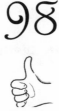

Use Protection

No glove, no love!

Did you know that an estimated 200–400 million people worldwide are infected with sexually transmitted diseases (STDs)? According to a national study done by the Centers for Disease Control and Prevention, 79.5 percent of college students have had sex. STDs occur most commonly in sexually active teenagers and young adults, especially those with multiple sex partners. Perhaps consequently, STDs are on the rise among college students. Most STDs can be successfully treated if they are diagnosed quickly enough. Here are some examples of common STDs:

- HIV/AIDS
- Genital warts
- Gonorrhea
- Syphilis
- Herpes
- Chlamydia
- Pubic lice or crabs
- Hepatitis

Left untreated, some STDs can have serious side effects such as sterility (being unable to have a child), brain damage, heart disease, birth defects, low birth weight and/or premature birth, increased risk for some types of cancer, and death.

You can help prevent the spread of STDs by:
- Practicing abstinence
- Only having sex with one person
- Using a condom every time
- Getting tested for stds regularly (one to two times per year)
- Alerting your partner that he or she needs to get tested too

Protect against HIV/AIDS

Fight against this attack on the body's immune system.

Acquired immune deficiency syndrome (AIDS) is the final, and most serious, stage of the human immunodeficiency virus (HIV), which causes severe damage to the immune system. AIDS was first recognized by the CDC in 1981, and today there are an estimated thirty-three million people worldwide who are infected with the disease.

Initial infection with HIV can produce no symptoms. Some people with the HIV infection remain without symptoms for years between the time they contract the virus and when they develop AIDS. However, other people experience flu-like symptoms with fever, rash, sore throat, and swollen lymph nodes approximately two weeks after contracting the virus. By the time AIDS develops, the cells of the immune system have been severely depleted by HIV, making the patient very susceptible to infection. Symptoms of this final stage of HIV infection are fever, night sweats, swollen glands, chills, weakness, and extreme weight loss. The symptoms of AIDS are primarily the result of infections, called opportunistic infections, which do not normally develop in individuals with healthy immune systems.

HIV can be transmitted through vaginal, anal, or oral sex with an infected person. It can also be transferred through the sharing of needles or from a mother to her child during pregnancy. Abstinence is the only 100 percent effective way to not contract HIV through sexual means. However, you can help slow the spread of HIV and AIDS by always using protection when having sex, avoiding drugs and needle sharing, and staying away from other people's blood, cuts, and wounds.

Visit www.aids.gov for more information.

100

Get a Pap Smear

A little smear goes a long way.

A Pap smear is a gynecological screening test that is used to detect cancerous processes in a woman's cervix. Abnormal findings can be investigated further or treated to possibly prevent cervical cancer. That's right, we can help prevent some cervical cancers!

You should have a Pap smear every year after becoming sexually active, especially because most women who contract human papillomavirus (HPV) become infected with the virus soon after becoming sexually active. Even if you have been vaccinated against HPV, you should get Pap smears annually because the vaccine does not prevent all forms of the virus that cause cancer.

Pap smears are ideally performed when you are not menstruating. At the appointment, your physician will insert a speculum into your vagina to gain access to your cervix. Cell samples are collected from the outer opening of the cervix using a small spatula, brush, or broom. The samples are then examined to determine if any abnormalities are present. Most test results are normal, but approximately 2–3 million abnormal Pap smear results are reported in the United States each year. If you're not convinced yet, check out these facts:

- Before the introduction of the Pap smear test, cervical cancer was a leading cause of death in women.

- Women who have never had a Pap smear are at higher risk for invasive cancers.
- Some 10–20 percent of cervical cancer cases occur in women who have not had a Pap smear in the preceding five years.
- As always, I want to help you prevent illness. Get tested! Check with your health-care provider about when you should have your Pap smear because the recommended frequency may be changing soon. Don't be afraid to spread eagle!

101

Take Charge of Your Colon Health

You only thought space was the final frontier.

The colon is often referred to as the sewer of the body. I know this sounds nasty, but your colon plays an important role in digestion by helping your body to expel waste. Ideally, you should be having several bowel movements each day, and you shouldn't be sitting on the toilet reading a magazine for twenty minutes each morning waiting for a small miracle to occur in your bathroom. Hello! Your bowel movements should occur fairly quickly after sitting down, and if they don't, you might be constipated.

Constipation is the slowed passage of digested food through your colon. Many things can cause this, including diet (lack of fiber), certain medications (narcotics such as codeine, oxycodone, and hydromorphone), iron supplements, aluminum-containing antacids, overuse of laxatives, hormone disorders, colon diseases, pelvic floor dysfunction, and habitual suppression of the urge to defecate. Why are you trying to hold that waste in? Stop it!

Some remedies for colon health can include eating plenty of fiber, low-fat foods, and more foods that are high in probiotics (lactobacillus acidophilus), which is healthy bacteria that's found in yogurt, milk, juices, and soy. Exercising and drinking more water are also important. I like sprinkling two tablespoons of flaxseed on top of oatmeal for breakfast. Some people find colonics, which were popularized by Dr. John Harvey Kellogg (the founder of Kellogg's cereal) from the 1900s to the 1940s, helpful also. Colonics may help prevent constipation, remove buildup in the colon, and improve overall health. This is important because buildup of fecal matter can prevent the absorption of water and nutrients, allow harmful bacteria and yeast to grow, and cause stagnant toxins to be absorbed into the bloodstream through the colon wall.

It's also important to know when it's more than constipation. Be sure to recognize the symptoms of colon cancer like constipation or diarrhea, blood in the stool, anemia, weight loss, pain in the lower abdomen, or intestinal obstruction. Talk to your doctor if you exhibit any of these symptoms. He or she may want to perform a colonoscopy, which is used to detect polyps and colon cancer.

102

Know the Risks for Testicular Cancer

Be aware of what's going on down there.

Testicular cancer is a rare disease that occurs when cells in one or both testicles become malignant. It accounts for only 1 percent of cancers in men of all ages. On average, about eight thousand men are diagnosed each year in the United States. Testicular cancer is impossible to prevent because some patients have no risk factors for the disease. However, early detection can save your life, and the best way to detect this deadly cancer early on is to know the risk factors.

Risk factors for developing testicular cancer:
- Any testicular abnormalities, including an undescended testicle or any abnormal development of the testicles
- Having a personal or family history of testicular cancer
- Having Klinefelter's syndrome, a genetic disorder that causes males to have an extra X chromosome

Make sure your doctor is aware if you have any of these risk factors.

Statistics show that men ages twenty to twenty-nine are most commonly affected by the disease. Most of the patients I have diagnosed have been younger men. Studies also show that Caucasian men develop testicular cancer at a higher rate than those of other races.

In addition to risk factors, you should also know the symptoms of testicular cancer, which may include a lump, swelling, or enlargement of the testicle or pain in the lower abdomen, back, or groin. If you notice any of these symptoms, consult your doctor. Diagnosis usually involves an ultrasound, blood tests, and a biopsy.

103

Maintain Breast Cancer Awareness

Feel your boobs; they're yours!

Breast cancer is an unpredictable disease that claims the life of one woman every thirteen minutes. Some people have no foreseeable risk for developing breast cancer and get it anyway, while other people appear to be high risk and never develop it. Because the disease is so hard to predict, you need to be aware of the risks and alert your doctor if you have any of them. Common risks for developing breast cancer include:

- Being female. Breast cancer can manifest in both men and women, but it is more common in women.
- Advanced age. Many people think the chance of getting breast cancer decreases with age but it actually increases.
- Personal history of breast cancer.
- Family history of breast cancer, especially in a female relative like your mother, grandmother, aunt, or sister.
- Giving birth to your first child after the age of thirty-five.
- Starting your period early in life or beginning menopause late in life.
- Obesity, alcohol, hormones, and previous radiation exposure.

Even if you don't have risk factors, you should watch for any changes in your breasts. Nobody is too young for breast cancer, so monthly self breast exams should be performed beginning in the teen years. This is important because most lumps are detected by the patient or their partner. More than 80 percent of lumps found in breasts are noncancerous, but they should always be tested to make sure. Regular mammograms are also imperative because the first signs of breast cancer usually show up on a mammogram before any lump can be seen. So do monthly self breast exams, get regular mammograms, and tell your health-care provider about any family history of breast cancer that you are aware of. Early detection gives patients the best chance for survival. Just ask any of the more than 1.7 million women who had breast cancer and are still alive today.

104

Get Your Hearing Checked

Say what?

It's important to have your hearing checked regardless of your age— it's not just the elderly who have trouble hearing! Experts say there are several causes of hearing loss, including occupational exposure (like with musicians and construction workers) and wax buildup in the external ear canal. Wax buildup is easily treated by using an over-the-counter wax remover, but unfortunately it goes unrecognized in 45 percent of patients. Just another reason to get your ears checked!

Early hearing loss detection and intervention is the first step to the successful treatment of any hearing problem. Hearing loss can be very subtle and develop gradually over many years, so often people with hearing impairment don't recognize it. Experts say that a loss of one or two decibels per year is not noticeable, but after ten to twenty years, that loss can seriously impair your ability to hear. Here are some symptoms of hearing loss that you should watch out for:

- Muffled hearing
- Difficulty understanding what people are saying, especially when there are competing voices or background noise
- Listening to the television or radio at very high volume
- Avoiding conversation and social interaction
- Pain, itching, hissing, or buzzing in the ear

If you notice these symptoms, it's definitely time to consult a doctor. If it turns out that you do need a hearing aid, don't get upset! Hearing aids aren't big and clunky objects anymore. They come in compact sizes that make them almost undetectable to the naked eye.

Hearing loss can be prevented by giving your ears a rest once in a while, wearing proper ear protection in loud areas, and limiting use of MP3 players, earphones, and headsets. Don't take your hearing for granted. I want you to be able to hear that big locomotive speeding toward you down the tracks!

105

Know How to Slow the Progression of COPD/Emphysema

Take care of your lungs—you only get two!

Emphysema is a lung disease that is characterized by an abnormal, permanent enlargement of air spaces distal to the terminal bronchioles. It occurs when the lung's internal structures are damaged and the tissue loses elasticity. It is often caused by exposure to toxic chemicals like those found in tobacco products. Did you hear that, smokers? The loss of elasticity causes air to become trapped in your lungs. Symptoms include shortness of breath, exhaustion, and/or an expanded chest.

If you are diagnosed with emphysema, the most important measure to slow its progression is for you to stop smoking (if you are a smoker) and avoid all exposure to tobacco smoke and lung irritants. If you quit smoking as soon as evidence of airway obstruction begins, you can significantly improve your prognosis. This also means absolutely no hanging around with smokers who insist on lighting up in your presence. Ever! You should also look into pulmonary rehabilitation, which can be very helpful in increasing your quality of life and teaching you how to actively manage your care. You must avoid air pollutants and people who are ill with respiratory problems because respiratory infections can be life-threatening to people with lung disease. You may also consider getting the influenza (flu) and pneumococcal pneumonia vaccinations, which have been shown to help prevent these infections. Check with your health-care provider about getting these shots. Good nutrition, including vitamin supplementation, may also mitigate emphysema symptoms. Regular aerobic exercise also builds up lung capacity and helps cleanse the lungs of stale air. Walking is an excellent choice; just avoid polluted areas.

Even if you don't have emphysema, you should talk with your health-care provider about how you can prevent damage to your lungs. Remember, you only get one pair in this lifetime. I hope you will choose to take excellent care of them. Don't smoke!

106

Watch Out for the Sweet and Salty

Sugar and spice and everything nice?

Our two greatest food cravings are for foods that are either sweet or salty. And heaven forbid, some of you are craving both! Crushing potato chips on top of your chocolate ice cream? You have just made a bad situation much worse!

The United States Department of Agriculture reports that the average American consumes anywhere from 150–170 pounds of simple sugar, also known as refined sugar, per year. Think about that—you just ate a whole person! This includes glucose, fructose, and sucrose. These refined sugars are depleted of these life forces: minerals, proteins, and vitamins. Did you know that four twelve-ounce cans of soda equals one-quarter pound of sugar? That's a lot of sugar! Some people drink four cans of soda a day.

Consuming too much sugar can lead to organ malfunction and hormone disruption. When these systems are disturbed and imbalanced, other pathological conditions manifest, including allergies, obesity, degenerative/organ disease, diabetes, depression, and behavioral problems. Is it any wonder that 60 percent of the American population is now considered overweight or obese?

So what can you do about it? Try to limit your intake of sugar and high fructose corn syrup (HFCS), which is a sweetener made from corn. In terms of composition, half of fructose syrup is nearly identical to table sugar (sucrose), which is composed of 50 percent fructose and 50 percent glucose. High fructose corn syrup is found in hot dogs, peanut butter, pickles, canned vegetables, applesauce, tomato soup, most sodas, and is even the first ingredient listed on a bottle of ranch dressing. Try to limit your intake of these things, and also watch out for doughnuts, cookies, cake, and ice cream. A great substitute is honey. You can also try swapping your dessert out with a piece of fruit. Or, if you must have some kind of dessert, split it with someone.

> *"Is tasteless food eaten without salt, or is there flavor in the white of an egg?"*
> —Job 6:6

Did you know that salt is produced through the evaporation of salt water and by mining? In ancient times, salt was such a precious commodity that it was traded ounce-for-ounce with gold. Most of us still use it every day, but it's important to limit your intake. Sodium is a required element for normal body function, so we shouldn't cut it out completely. Typically, you should have between 2,200 and 3,000 mg of salt a day.

Salt is a preservative, so it's found in almost everything we eat, including hot sauce, dill pickles, chips, sweets, and ice cream. I know in Matthew 5:13, God said that we were the salt of the Earth. He did not tell you to personally eat all of the salt on the Earth! So, you say, "Oh, I have a sweet tooth." Now what? You're going to tell me that you have a salty tooth, too? To limit your salt intake, don't salt your food before you taste it, understand food labels, and make sure you're taking in less than 3,000 mg of salt per day. Overall, choose a diet that is low in salt. The salt patrol is looking for you—leave the salt shaker on the table!

107

Don't Underestimate the Importance of Laughter

"The most wasted of all days is one without laughter."
—E.E. Cummings

When was the last time you laughed until you cried and had to hold your sides? If you can't remember, it's been far too long! Did you know that when you laugh, your brain releases neurochemicals called endorphins? These feel-good chemicals make you feel great and reduce feelings of depression considerably. A few good laughs can release enough endorphins to turn your whole day around. Since you are planning on living until you are 131 years old, you will definitely need more than just a few good laughs to make those years enjoyable!

"He will yet fill your mouth with laughter
and your lips with shouts of joy."
—Job 8:21

There is an old saying that goes "Take time to stop and smell the roses." Here are your new instructions: take time to slow down and laugh more! Sometime when you are in a drugstore, take ten minutes and go to the card section. Read the cards just for fun and see how many laughs you get! You'll be shocked at how much better you feel when you leave the store. It's fun and free, so why not give it a try? Try going to a comedy club, watching a funny movie (I love Tyler Perry!), and staying connected with funny friends who make you laugh. Also, spend time with your children or grandchildren. Nothing brightens up your day more than spending time with these miniature comedians. There's something so refreshingly honest and light-hearted about the way children see the world. Be childlike yourself when you can't spend time with children. Try to get back in that state of mind once in a while—the benefits are overwhelming.

"Laughter is the shortest distance between two people."
—Victor Borge

"Laughter gives us distance. It allows us to step back from an event, deal with it, and then move on."
—Bob Newhart

108

Avoid Asbestos

Asbestos poisoning can be fatal.

Asbestos is well recognized as a health hazard, and conse-quently it is highly regulated. However, an estimated 1.3 million employees in the construction industry still have significant asbestos exposure at work. The heaviest exposures occur from the removal of asbestos during renovation or demolition. Individuals are also likely to be exposed during the manufacturing of asbestos products (like textiles, friction products, insulation, and other building materials) and during automotive brake and clutch repair work.

When asbestos fibers are inhaled, most fibers are expelled, but some can become lodged in the lungs and remain there throughout your entire life. Over time, fibers accumulate and cause scarring and inflammation. Enough scarring and inflammation can affect breathing, leading to disease and even cancer-related death (such as lung cancer). When it comes to asbestos, prevention is key because it can take many years for the damage to become apparent.

You can limit exposure by wearing protective gear if you are working in the construction industry, having your home tested for asbestos, and not handling any products or materials containing high amounts of it. If you're not able to fully avoid asbestos, watch out for these symptoms of hazardous levels of exposure:

- Shortness of breath
- Chronic cough
- Chest pain
- Difficulty breathing
- Abnormal chest X-ray

If you have been exposed to asbestos and are experiencing any of these or related asbestos symptoms, you should seek medical attention as soon as possible.

For more information, visit the Environmental Protection Agency's website at www.epa.gov.

109

Avoid Lead Poisoning

Don't let lead destroy your health!

Did you know that the United States didn't stop using lead paint until 1978, fifty years after European countries? Since then, lead poisoning has become much less of a health threat. However, if you work around lead, you could still be at significant risk of suffering from mild to moderate lead poisoning. Unborn babies, infants, and young children are especially at risk because exposure to even very small amounts can lead to permanent damage. Lead poisoning is still one of the most overlooked child epidemics in America and the most chronic environmental illness affecting children.

It's impossible to eliminate all exposure to lead because it's something that occurs naturally in our environment. The truth is that every living creature is exposed to small amounts of lead through household dust, lead-based paint, food, drinking water, air, soil, and a variety of products we buy and use. What we can do to protect ourselves against lead poisoning is minimize our exposure to it.

How you can minimize exposure to lead:
- Don't wear outdoor shoes indoors; you may bring lead in on the bottom of your feet.

- Give your pets' feet, legs, and undersides a good rubdown with a coarse towel after taking them outdoors for the same reason.
- Wash your children's hands on a regular basis.
- Wash children's toys often.
- Buy American-made products. Not only is it good for the economy, but it is safer, too. Many countries where goods are produced do not have lead laws like ours.

110

Be Healthy When You Travel

So you're going on vacation? That's so wonderful!
Remember to pack your meds!

Everyone needs to get away once in a while; a vacation is good for your body, mind, and soul. And I'm sure you've got everything you need in those suitcases, right? Wrong! Some-times it's the most obvious things we forget when we are getting ready to go out of town—our driver's license, passport, or plane tickets. Even worse, my patients frequently leave on trips and forget their medications. This can potentially be very dangerous depending on what medications you take on a daily basis, especially if you take something like insulin or heart medications.

When you leave town or know you're going to be away from home for an extended period of time, always bring extra medication with you. What if you get stranded at the airport? This is especially important if you're asthmatic and frequently need an inhaler. If you can't carry your bottles with you, be sure to copy your prescriptions or bottle labels, and carry those with you in case you are hurt and can't speak for yourself. Don't get pulled over and have to explain to the police officer what the pills in your cup holder are for! Keep your medications labeled and with you at all times.

If you are going out of the country, be sure to notify your health-care provider well in advance to see if you need any inoculations or medications before your trip, such as medication for malaria. Also, be sure to ask about the safety of drinking the water where you are going. For instance, if you visit Mexico, it would be wise to not drink the water. It contains bacteria that your body isn't used to, and it may cause diarrhea, which will deplete your electrolytes. This can dehydrate you and possibly make you very ill. That doesn't sound like a very fun vacation, does it?

Important:

Be sure to notify airlines in advance if you require insulin and will be bringing it with you on an airplane. Airlines have strict rules about what liquids you can bring onboard, and you don't want any surprises.

111

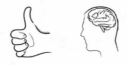

Have a Date Night with Yourself

I don't care if you're single, married, widowed, divorced, or shacking up, you're probably the best date you've had in a long time!

Let's face it, a romantic evening with the perfect man or woman isn't in the cards for everyone. There isn't always going to be someone wonderful around to make you feel warm and fuzzy. So my advice is to turn off your cell phone, get in the car, and go out on a date with yourself. Yes, I'm serious! What are you afraid of? Go out to dinner at that nice restaurant you've wanted to try, or go see that new movie alone! Go to the matinee for cheaper prices and to avoid the crowds. Treat yourself to some of that delicious movie theater popcorn (without all that salt and butter, of course). Nobody knows you like you do, so instead of going out on a boring date, plan that special and exciting date that you know you would like for yourself. Go get a massage or a manicure and pedicure (girl, your feet are looking and feeling rough!), go golfing, or take up piano lessons. Whatever you decide to do, don't let anyone interrupt you. On my date night, my response to people who are trying to burden me with unnecessary questions and tasks is either "I don't know" or "I don't care."

I am definitely not afraid to go out alone. I am constantly being invited to different gatherings, but I am a woman who enjoys her alone time. Me time gives me the chance to clear out all the clutter in my mind. Plus, when I go to restaurants alone, I am usually treated much better than when I go with a crowd. I like dealing with people one-on-one, and when I have the chance to speak with my waiter, address him by name, and get to know him a little bit, somehow my order always comes out faster, hotter, and exactly the way I wanted it! A little kindness goes a long way. So instead of worrying about finding a date for this weekend, try taking yourself out for a night on the town or quiet evening at home. You won't regret it! You can always go out with that new girl or guy next weekend. And don't go out driving through a fast-food restaurant loading up on fried foods and biscuits singing, "Praise God, from whom all blessings flow!" Strawberry jelly please!

112

Get a Physical

When was the last time you had one?

The US Preventative Services Task Force has done away with recommendations for healthy people getting physicals. How often you should get one is dependent upon not only your health but also your age and, of course, on your insurance coverage or ability to pay for one. Those who are advanced in age and/or have specific health concerns should consult with their doctors about their personal needs.

At the very least, young women should have a gynecological exam once yearly after they become sexually active or starting at the age of eighteen, whichever comes first. Sometimes a general practitioner can provide both a yearly physical and a gynecological exam at the same time so women don't have to go to two checkups every year.

There are variations on recommendations for men and women in their twenties, so check with your health-care provider. While not a requirement, many doctors still recommend you get a physical every three years or so, while others suggest you need only two physicals in your twenties. Naturally, if you are at risk for medical conditions and/or have an illness or a family history of early onset illnesses, you may want to get a physical more frequently.

Between the ages of forty and sixty-five, it may be more important to have a physical every two years or more often if you are at risk for developing other medical conditions. Women should begin having mammograms every one or two years in their forties. People sixty-five and older should ideally get a physical once yearly to continue to check for development of diseases and overall health. Men need to be sure to get tested for prostate cancer. After age fifty, both men and women should begin having yearly rectal exams to assess risk for colorectal cancer. When I have to give my male patients a rectal exam, they say, "Oh no, Dr. Walker! Not again!" I tell them, "Trust me, this is hurting me more than it is you. . . . Now, bottoms up!" Check with your provider to find out what's best for you.

113

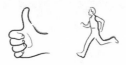

Take a Vacation

Everyone needs to get away.

Taking a vacation gives you time to relax and enjoy yourself while being free from your everyday responsibilities at home and at the office. I always say I'd love to see the glaciers in Alaska but only if they'll bring them to me. Honestly, I'm more of a beach girl. No matter where you go, vacations can give you some unforgettable memories that will last a lifetime. Making happy memories is good for the soul, don't you agree? Vacations allow you to enjoy an escape from reality, become physically and spiritually more in tune, and come home with a better mental outlook. They also give you something to look forward to! Here are my tips for the perfect vacation:

- Make sure you have a vacation budget. Nothing like being broke on day two of your trip!
- Give your boss and colleagues plenty of advance notice that you're leaving.
- Reserve your flights and hotels early.
- Pack light.
- Enjoy the planning and packing as part of the overall experience.
- Leave your phone and laptop at home.

- Don't use your vacation as an excuse to drink excessively.
- Have your sunscreen readily available, regardless of the weather conditions at your destination.
- Take a good book and catch up on your reading.
- Make friends and stay in touch with them once you return home.
- Take plenty of pictures so you have a reminder when it's a dreary day in the office.
- Remember to pack your sunglasses to block those harmful UV rays.

Studies show that taking a vacation can make you feel more relaxed and more focused when you return. Vacations can also reduce stress, which may lead to a longer life in general.

Bon voyage! (That's French, darling. . . .)

114

Cook in Cast-Iron Pots and Skillets

A super easy solution to iron deficiency.

The body needs iron in the blood to carry oxygen from the lungs to the rest of the body. However, it has been estimated that only 65–70 percent of Americans get enough iron. Low iron levels mean that the blood does not efficiently circulate oxygen, which causes a feeling of tiredness and sometimes headaches. Extreme iron deficiency can cause anemia.

Cooking in cast iron is known to greatly increase the dietary source of iron. This is especially true when cooking foods high in acid, such as tomato-based sauces. As you might expect, frequent stirring of food will also increase the amount of iron. There is less of an effect for foods that are quickly fried in the skillet. My grandma cooked in cast-iron skillets, and my family still uses them today!

Did you know that it's also possible to have too much iron onboard, which can lead to toxicity? However, in an average diet, it is highly unlikely that cooking with cast iron will bring a person to this level. Most people who achieve toxicity overdose on iron supplements. For this reason, you should always consult your health-care provider before taking any iron supplements.

In addition to cooking in cast iron, try these iron-rich foods to boost your levels of this vital element:

- Beef
- Spinach
- Dried fruit
- Clams and oysters
- Chicken and pork liver
- Sardines (a rich source of calcium and omega 3 too!)

115

Prevent Asthma-Related Death

Breathing is important—make sure you can do it!

There are nearly 1.7 million ER visits due to asthma in the United States each year. It is estimated that approximately 22.9 million Americans have asthma, an inflammatory disorder of the airways that causes attacks of wheezing, shortness of breath, chest tightness, and coughing. Each year, there are more than four thousand deaths due to asthma, and asthma is indicated as a contributing factor in nearly seven thousand other deaths. Many of these deaths could've been avoided with proper treatment and care. If you are asthmatic, stay away from areas with bad air quality and don't ever let anyone smoke in your house—especially you! Not smoking is particularly important for asthmatics because their lung function already declines faster than normal. So the answer is: don't smoke! Make your lungs last a lifetime.

It's important to know and avoid your own asthmatic triggers, but here are some common ones to watch for:

- Animals (pet hair or dander).
- Changes in weather (most often cold weather triggers asthma).
- Chemicals in the air or in food.

- Extended periods of exercise—you can exercise if you have asthma, but you may need to take breaks during workouts or take medication before exercising. Check with your doctor.
- Stressful situations.
- Dust, mold, and pollen in the air.
- Respiratory infections, such as the common cold.
- Tobacco smoke.
- Excrement and debris from decomposing bugs, which are small enough to be inhaled. Call pest control!

If you have asthma, never leave home without your inhaler, and ask your doctor what to do in the event of an asthma attack. You should also ask your doctor about flu and pneumonia shots. I am still seeing too many untimely deaths due to asthma; please don't be another one.

116

Help Slow Global Warming

"It's getting hot in here!"
—Nelly

When sunlight reaches Earth's surface, a small amount of it is absorbed to warm the planet, while the rest is radiated back to the atmosphere. The atmosphere then reflects back heat energy, which is what we call the "Greenhouse Effect." The higher the concentration of greenhouse gases like carbon dioxide in the atmosphere, the more heat energy is reflected back to Earth and the hotter Earth gets. Global warming is the term used to describe a gradual increase in the average temperature of the Earth's atmosphere and its oceans. It's a change that is believed to be permanently altering the Earth's climate. The increased volumes of carbon dioxide and other greenhouse gases released by the burning of fossil fuels, land clearing, agriculture, and other human activities are thought to be the primary sources of global warming.

Over the past one hundred years, the average temperature of the Earth has risen between 0.4 and 0.8 degrees Celsius. Scientists have recently predicted that average global temperatures could increase between 1.4 and 5.8 degrees by the year 2100. The scientific consensus is that global warming is a very real threat to our planet. Changes resulting from global warming could be detrimental and may include rising sea levels due to the melting of polar ice and an increase in storms and other severe weather events.

Seven things you can do to help the environment:

- Copy Portland, Oregon, and use energy-efficient light bulbs.
- Drive environmentally friendly cars.
- Don't overuse your air conditioner during hot months.
- Avoid opening the refrigerator unnecessarily during the day.
- Buy green products.
- Go organic: Try eating only organic fruits and veggies. Plant that garden!
- Buy products packaged with recycled materials.

Who knows what could happen if we all do our part?

117

Keep a First-Aid Kit on Hand

Know where it is, what's in it, and how to use it.

This might seem like common sense, but having a first-aid kit handy has the potential to save lives in the event of an emergency. Something simple like an aspirin, a bandage, or a bit of alcohol can be very important in a crisis. Things like extra EpiPens, inhalers, blankets, and bottled water can also be useful and should be included when possible. Keep a small kit in your car, and include water and extra blankets during cold months. Every home should have a first-aid kit, too. Keep it in a central location that everyone can access easily.

Kits should be fully stocked with at least the following supplies:

- Bandages: Have bandages in assorted sizes—everything from the tiny finger bandages to the big square style. Your kit should also include big gauze bandages in various shapes and sizes and a roll of gauze bandaging.
- Medical tape: Designed to be used on skin, medical tape is perfect for attaching gauze bandages to skin. It also works when you need to tape together a quick finger splint.
- Medical scissors: These generally have blunt tips so they can be used against skin without risk of puncture. You'll need them to cut medical tape or to cut bandages to appropriate sizes.

- Alcohol wipes: You can buy these individually wrapped. Use them to sterilize and clean wounds, scrapes, and scratches.
- Peroxide: This is used medically for cleaning wounds, removing dead tissue, and rinsing the mouth.
- Triple antibiotic ointment: This combination of bacitracin, neomycin, and polymyxin B topical (for the skin) is used to treat and prevent infections in minor cuts, scrapes, or burns on your skin.

Remember, serious injuries that require medical attention should be taken care of as soon as possible. First-aid is great for small injuries, but it's always better to be safe than sorry.

118

Guard against Staph Infections

*Bad boy, bad boy! Whatcha gonna
do when they come for you?*

Staph (staphylococcus aureus) is a potentially life-threatening bacterium that lives on the skin, especially around the mouth, nose, and genital area. Everybody carries the bacteria, but most never become sick. However, if the skin is broken due to injury, the bacteria can penetrate the wound and cause infection in the skin, blood, bones, and lungs. People with weakened immune systems are at a higher risk for staph infection. Over the past fifty years, some staph bacteria have become resistant to antibiotics like penicillin, making them particularly dangerous.

You are most at risk for getting a staph infection if you are diabetic, immunocompromised, have an indrilling foreign body, or suffer frequent or chronic disruptions to the skin. Common symptoms include boils and redness near a wound.

Ways to prevent a staph infection:
- Staph infections occur when the bacteria enter an open wound, so clean and cover cuts. People with open cuts or injuries should keep wounds covered with a bandage at all times.
- Report any oozing, redness, or puss from a wound to your doctor. Staph infections can get ugly.

- Wash your hands often.
- Use clean razors. Some people habitually share razors or combs—this is a no-no! Using another person's comb, brush, towel, or razor can greatly increase your risk of infection.
- Don't share toothbrushes.
- If you get a tattoo, research tattoo artists and check the cleanliness of their shops before making a selection.

119

Prevent Arthritis

Old man Arthur is your new best friend!

A crippling condition characterized by stiffness, joint pain, difficulty walking, and swelling, osteoarthritis is a progressive degenerative disease that generally gets worse as you age. However, arthritis affects people of all ages, including at least three hundred thousand children. Today, more than 45 million people in the United States suffer from arthritis, and it is the second leading cause of work-related disability. Trying to prevent arthritis is preferable to trying to treat the pain that comes with this condition. Crippling arthritis can cause chronic pain that can lead to depression, social isolation, and dangerous falls that may result in bone fracture.

How to help prevent osteoarthritis:
- Learn how to relax. Tense muscles apply stress to a joint.
- Practice good posture and always bend your knees when lifting heavy objects. Never lift from your back.
- Protect your joints. Wear warm, protective clothing in cold weather.
- Maintain healthy calcium and vitamin D levels.
- Maintain a healthy weight.
- Avoid soft chairs and sleep on a firm mattress.

- Soak in a hot tub, especially after strenuous exercise.
- Stretch and exercise!

Fact:

The bromelain in pineapple can ease the pain of arthritis.

120

Lower High Blood Pressure (Hypertension)

It's a silent killer.

Your heart is a pump, and when it contracts or beats it sends blood through your blood vessels, which increases pressure. Blood pressure is a force that is exerted on the walls of your arteries as blood flows through them. This is the systolic pressure, or the top number of your pressure. The pressure decreases when your heart relaxes between beats. This is your diastolic pressure, or the bottom number. Blood pressure is determined by the amount of blood your heart pumps and the amount of resistance to blood flow in your arteries. So the more blood your heart pumps and the narrower your arteries, the higher your pressure will be. Symptoms of high blood pressure may include a dull headache, dizzy spells, or nose bleeds.

The two types of high blood pressure are primary (or essential) and secondary hypertension. Primary hypertension is the most common and has no identifiable cause. Secondary hypertension develops in less than 10 percent of people and usually has an identifiable cause such as kidney disease or illegal drug use. Risk factors include age (it increases as you get older), race (it's common among African-American), family history, being overweight, lack of physical activity, smoking those nasty cigarettes, too much salt (which causes fluid retention), heavy drinking, stress, and conditions such as high cholesterol, diabetes, and sleep apnea. Consult your physician to determine what your ideal blood pressure should be.

Ways to lower your pressure:
- Lose weight, exercise, and reduce stress.
- Begin a low-fat, low-salt diet and reduce alcohol intake.
- Don't smoke.

And listen to your doctor! I often have problems getting my patients to take their blood pressure medication, especially the men. They say the medicines make them impotent, and they look and feel so good without the meds that they don't see why they should take them. Well, I tell them, you're gonna look good in a coffin, too! Keep in mind that most people with high blood pressure have few or no symptoms at all until they have a heart attack or stroke.

121

Try More Resveratrol

Your wine list, please. . . .

Even though the French tend to eat a diet high in fat, they actually have a low incidence of heart disease. Many believe this can be traced to their frequent consumption of red wine. Red wine has anticoagulating effects that may help guard against heart disease, but that's not all. Many feel that resveratrol, an antioxidant contained in red wine, may also play a role.

One of the best food sources for resveratrol in its natural state is peanuts. They have a significantly higher resveratrol content than even the berries and grapes that produce the wine! Even though a lot of research is still being done on this product, preliminary studies suggest that resveratrol may be an excellent antioxidant that can help reduce memory loss, ward off viruses, and act as an excellent antiaging cure.

Resveratrol, I've got my eye on you!

122

Keep Your Urinary Tract Healthy

Urinary tract infections are no fun!

A urinary tract infection is an infection that begins in your urinary system, which includes your kidneys, ureters, bladder, and the urethra. Any part of your urinary system can get infected, but most infections develop in the lower urinary tract area (the urethra and bladder). While a urinary tract infection in your bladder can be painful, serious consequences can occur if the infection spreads to your kidneys.

Urinary tract infections occur when bacteria enters your urinary tract through the urethra and begins to multiply in the bladder. Your urinary system is designed to keep out this bacteria, but it doesn't always succeed. Urinary tract infections can usually be treated with antibiotics, so see your doctor if you think you may have one. Women are more likely than men to suffer from urinary tract infections, so they need to be particularly careful. Here are some things you can do to aid in preventing an uncomfortable infection:

- Practice good hygiene habits. Clean the area around your vagina and rectum daily. Always wipe this area from front to back to prevent bacteria from entering the urethra or vagina.

- Drink half your body weight (in ounces) in water every day. Cranberry juice is also beneficial in the prevention of urinary tract infections.
- Urinate before and after sex to help keep bacteria out of your genital area.
- Avoid excessive use of products that can be irritating to your genitals, such as vaginal douches and some feminine hygiene products.
- Don't try to hold urine in all day. Go when you have to go! When my family and I were on the country roads and had to go, we simply used nature's bathroom.

123

Protect against Osteoporosis

*The human body has 206 bones; keep
every one of yours healthy!*

Osteoporosis occurs over time as your bone tissue thins and your bones lose their density. There are no symptoms of the disease in its early stages. Many times a patient won't even know they have osteoporosis until they break a bone. Wrist, hip, and spine fractures are most common, but this disease does not discriminate—all of your bones are at risk when you have osteoporosis.

Although women are four times more likely to develop osteoporosis, men are also at risk. Isn't it funny how we usually associate things like breast cancer, menopause, and osteoporosis with women, only to discover that men can also develop these diseases and conditions? Besides being female, other risk factors include age (the older you are, the more likely you are to be affected), race (Caucasians, Asians, and Latinos are at the highest risk), family history, being thin, having a personal history of broken bones, being menopausal, having a low count of estrogen in women or testosterone in men, and vitamin C or D deficiency. Smoking, alcohol abuse, and certain medications can also contribute to bone loss. Because osteoporosis can't be diagnosed in the early stages, it's vital that you work to prevent it. The National Osteoporosis Foundation recommends these five steps to keep bones healthy and prevent osteoporosis:

- Eat right. Get your daily recommended amounts of calcium and vitamin D.
- Exercise. Engage in regular weight-bearing and muscle strengthening workouts.
- Maintain a healthy lifestyle and weight. Avoid smoking and excessive alcohol consumption.
- Talk to your health-care provider about bone health.
- Get tested. Have a bone density test and take medication when appropriate. Ask your health-care provider about your options regarding these medications.

124

Ward Off Pneumonia

Guess what? Grandma was right—
chicken noodle soup helps!

Did you know that pneumonia kills more people in the United States each year than all other vaccine-preventable diseases combined? An infection of the lungs, pneumonia can be caused by many different organisms, including bacteria, viruses, parasites, and fungi. The severity of the disease depends on the type of organism causing the pneumonia as well as your age and underlying health. It can range from mild to severe and, in some cases, can even be deadly. Health-care workers or those suffering from chronic disease are especially at risk. Here are some steps you can take to prevent the disease:

- Wash hands frequently, especially after eating, using the restroom, coughing, being outside, or coming into contact with sick people.
- Don't smoke—it damages your lungs' ability to ward off infection.
- Exercise daily to increase lung function. Get walking!
- Drink water and eat a healthy diet full of nutrient-rich fruits and vegetables.
- Ask your health-care provider about the pneumonia vaccine and annual flu shot.

- Also check with your health-care provider about the Hib vaccine for your children—it helps prevent pneumonia caused by haemophilus influenzae type b in kids.

You should also know and watch out for the main symp-toms of pneumonia, which are: cough with greenish or yellow mucus and/or bloody sputum, fever with shaking chills, sharp or stabbing chest pain worsened by deep breathing or coughing, and rapid, shallow breathing.

125

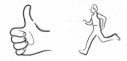

Enjoy Some Sexual Healing

What happens in your bedroom, stays in your bedroom.

Having plenty of good sex with your spouse is a fun and healthy way to live until you are 131 years old! According to the Bible, it is a blessing to have sexual relations with your spouse, and it's also important to sustain a certain level of intimacy in your marriage. And think of all those calories you're burning—now that's what I call multitasking!

> *"Marriage should be honored by all, and the marriage bed kept pure."*
> —*Hebrews 13:4*

> *"The husband should fulfill his marital duty to his wife, and likewise the wife to her husband."*
> —*1 Corinthians 7:3*

See, there's nothing to be ashamed of; it's not a sin!

According to research at the University of North Carolina, kissing and hugging both raise your levels of oxytocin, a hormone commonly associated with bonding and love. Scottish researchers have stated that having sex on a regular basic lowers anxiety, stress, and blood pressure levels. So if you're feeling a little stressed out, you know what to do! And don't start pulling that hoodoo voodoo on your spouse to try and make a point. Withholding sex from your partner isn't going to solve anything!

Ladies, don't ever stop dating your husband, and husbands don't ever stop dating your wife. Men, ladies enjoy when you put on your nice boxers (or briefs) and good cologne at bedtime. We don't want to see you at the foot of the bed in those old, raggedy shorts from back in the day, saying things like, "Big Poppa's comin' atcha!" Let's try something a little more romantic, OK? And ladies, don't get lazy and start coming to bed with face cream on, big pink rollers in your hair, and that flannel gown, batting your eyes at your husband! I'm sure he's going to say, "Not tonight dear, I have a headache." Gentlemen prefer black lace.

126

Know the Signs of Seasonal Affective Disorder

Smiling all summer and whining all winter?

Seasonal affective disorder (SAD) is a type of depression that occurs around the same time every year. Most people with seasonal affective disorder develop symptoms in the fall that may continue through the entire winter. Common symptoms include depleted energy levels and feeling moody, sad, and unstable.

It seems that SAD develops from inadequate bright light during the winter months. For this reason, the incidences of SAD increase in people who are living farther away from the equator. Studies also show that it is less common where there is snow on the ground. It's possible but much more rare for SAD to cause depression in the spring or summer months instead. People of all ages and both genders can develop the disorder, but women tend to suffer from it more frequently.

You may have seasonal affective disorder if you experience a deep sadness or depression that affects your everyday life during certain times of the year. Every time the leaves start to fall, I see a lot of seasonal affective disorder. Seeking professional help for this condition can greatly increase your quality of life and help to keep your mood stable throughout the year. Treatment for the "winter blues" or the "hibernation reaction" can include psychotherapy, light therapy (phototherapy), and/or medication.

127

Watch Your Cholesterol Levels

Keep the good (HDL) high and the bad (LDL) low.

Cholesterol is a soft, waxy substance that's made in your liver and can also be found in some foods. It's stored in your blood and cells and helps your body make hormones (including sex hormones), acts as a precursor to vitamin D, and makes the bile acids that aid in digestion.

There are two types of cholesterol: HDL and LDL. HDL (high-density lipoprotein) is "good" cholesterol that helps your body by carrying cholesterol away from the arteries to your liver. High HDL reduces your risk of heart disease. LDL (low-density lipoprotein) is "bad" cholesterol. Too much LDL can build up on your artery walls and harden, forming plaque. This increases your risk of heart disease.

Ideally, your total cholesterol level should be less than 200 mg/dl. Optimal HDL cholesterol levels are 60 mg/dl and over, though 40–59 mg/dl is considered acceptable. Optimal LDL levels are less than 100 mg/dl, but they're not considered borderline high until 130–159 mg/dl. There aren't any symptoms of high cholesterol, so ask your health-care provider if you should get checked.

The two reasons people have high cholesterol are family and food. For most people, the cause of their high cholesterol is consumption of too much of certain types of fats. Foods that are high in saturated fats and trans fats can raise your LDL, or "bad" cholesterol, levels. Remember, cholesterol comes from animals—there is no cholesterol in fruits or vegetables. Two popular foods that have the highest of high cholesterol levels are egg yolks and liver. Other sources are rib meat, butter, cheese, and whole milk. Certain shellfish like shrimp can also have high cholesterol, and duck and goose skin are both culprits.

Eating foods that are high in cholesterol is only part of the equation because genetics also plays a role. However, food consumption is the part of the equation that you can control, so try to limit anything with high cholesterol levels.

128

Eat More Soy

Behold the power of soy.

Sometimes referred to as greater bean or edamame, the soybean is a species of annual legume that is native to east Asia. This exotic plant has been used in China for over five thousand years, mainly to add nitrogen to the soil during crop rotation. Today, we know that soy has a lot of potential health benefits.

The FDA has approved soy as an official cholesterol-lowering food, stating that 25 mg per day as part of a low cholesterol and saturated fat diet may reduce the risk of heart disease. This is because it contains a group of plant estrogens (phytoestrogens) called isoflavones, which are believed to have protective health benefits. Soy also contains high levels of phytic acid, which may reduce risk for cancer, diabetes, and inflammation. Studies have shown soy to aid in reducing the risk of heart disease, osteoporosis, and some cancers. It may also help relieve some common symptoms of menopause, such as hot flashes, night sweats, and mood swings. Pass the soy, ladies!

The main producers of soy are the United States, Brazil, Argentina, China, and India. Soy foods are everywhere. You can buy anything from soy nuts and chips to beverages and desserts. Incorporating these products into your diet is an easy and natural way to do something good for your health, especially since soy is also a great source of vitamins! The water-soluble vitamins in soybeans are thiamine, riboflavin, niacin, pantothenic acid, biotin, folic acid, inositol, and choline. Fat-soluble vitamins present in the soybean are vitamins A and E.

Research on soy continues to prove its role in prevention and treatment of disease. It can be considered one of nature's healthiest and highest quality food sources. My favorite soy snack is soy nuts—I open the bag and eat them all up! They are also great with a salad. Yum!

129

Participate in Medical Research

Learn how you can help to find a cure.

Most people don't understand the importance medical research plays in our lives. Stop and think for a moment about how different the world would be if we didn't have vaccines for diseases like polio and smallpox or medications to treat high blood pressure, glaucoma, or the common cold. We tend to take much of our health care for granted and often forget the history behind our modern-day vaccines, medications, treatments, and cures. For example, did you know the hypodermic syringe was invented way back in 1850 by Charles Pravaz and Alexander Wood?

Medical research has led to the development of vaccines for rabies, polio, smallpox, diphtheria, and measles/mumps/rubella. When we began to understand the relationship between electricity and physiology, it led to the development of the EKG (electrocardiograph), EEG (electroencephalograph), and several other technologies that analyze the body using electricity. Eventually, this led to the invention of the MRI (magnetic resonance imaging) machine by Paul Lauterbur and Peter Mansfield. Isn't that amazing? These technologies have become an integral part of how we diagnose and treat diseases today. As a doctor, I can't imagine a world without the EKG!

Medical research in fields such as physics and chemistry are still extremely important in the development of modern-day medicine. Today, we are facing a rise in communicable diseases such as HIV, hepatitis, influenza, and West Nile virus. Medical and clinical research continues to seek cures for these and many other germ-based diseases. You can help by participating in medical research studies in your area and donating to funds that sponsor research. Many people find it rewarding to donate to causes that research cures for specific diseases that their loved one suffers from or died because of. So let's continue to unravel the mysteries of the universe together! OK, captain!

130

Give, Give, Give.

God was a giver; He gave us His only son.

Cheap! Stingy! Chintzy! Oh, my goodness . . . these are some of the worst traits in the world. You're basically telling God, "I don't trust you enough to give, tithe at church, help a person in need, or donate to a charitable organization. It might not come back to me tenfold." But God says, "I'll open up the windows of heaven and pour you out a blessing you won't have room enough to receive."

So stop being so tight-fisted and follow the five golden keys of generosity:

- Don't be greedy—keep the great advice your momma gave you and give away the rest!
- Give your time. Time is one of the hardest things for us to give up. Money changes hands easily, but giving someone your time says that you are there to listen, that you care, and that you want to help.
- Give to your church. Churches help so many people in so many different ways. Giving to your church each week will help spread the love around.

- Don't expect anything in return. You'll never be disappointed! Giving is not about receiving.
- Give your patience, kindness, and love.

One charity that I'm particularly fond of was started by Paul Crouch and his beautiful wife, Jan (founders of TBN, the Trinity Broadcasting Network). Their Second Chance program provides religious texts and inspiration to two million inmates throughout the United States. To contribute to this excellent program, visit www.tbn.org.

"The King will reply, 'I tell you the truth, whatever you did for one of the least of these brothers of mine, you did for.'"
Matthew 25:40

131

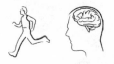

Go Out and Play!

Playtime isn't just for kids anymore.

When was the last time you took some time out to just relax, enjoy yourself, and play? And I don't mean going out for happy hour at the bar with the girls, guzzling wine. What about taking your kids to the park and running, leaping, and jumping right along with them? Taking time to see the world through a child's eyes again can be a deep experience that transforms you. I know that sometimes when my hectic schedule and personal life get to be a little too much, I need time to go out into the world and play again. I play with my Barbie dolls, go to the zoo or the aquarium, or put on a tiara and pretend I'm a princess for the day. Yes, you heard me right!

It was easy to be happy when you were a child, wasn't it? Sure you got upset and cried once in a while, but the things that you allowed to get to you then were a far cry from some of the stuff on your plate these days. Allow yourself to let go of whatever's troubling you for a little while, and return to that happy childhood state of mind. God gave you an imagination; you might as well use it!

There are so many ways for you to play. Why not try soccer, softball, basketball, or tetherball? Remember recess? Most kids say recess is their favorite "subject" in school anyway! If you're not into sports, grab some friends and take a short road trip for the weekend, go hunting for treasures at a flea market, or bake a low-fat cake and throw yourself a party just for fun. Invite your girlfriends over and have a pajama party. Stay up all night long playing games, laughing, and having a ball! I make my life exciting and fun every day, regardless of what else is going on. It's not always easy, but it is well worth the effort to make playtime a part of your daily routine. The benefits of play include decreased stress, increased relaxation, and better sleep. Plus, you burn calories, too! I play hard because I get a good return on my investment. Remember, everyone deserves to play!

Can you come out and play with me?

About the Author

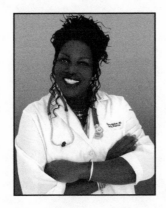

Dr. Valerie Walker is a family-medicine physician originally from McIntyre, Georgia. She graduated with an MD from Temple University in Philadelphia and completed her internship and residency at Medical College of Georgia in Augusta. Dr. Walker is now the medical director of the Dr. Valerie Walker Medical Center in St. Louis, where she practices holistic, traditional, and spiritual healing methods on over six thousand patients.

Walker is an in-demand public speaker who tours nation-wide, captivating her audiences with her wit, knowledge, and humor. She hosts her own TV show, *House Calls with Dr. Valerie Walker*, and her hobbies include playing the piano and electric bass and collecting Barbie dolls.

For more information about Dr. Valerie Walker, visit www.DrValerieWalker.com.